MIX
Papier aus verantwortungsvollen Quellen
Paper from responsible sources
FSC® C105338

Anuj Singh Parihar

Host Modulation in Periodontology

Anchor Academic
Publishing

Parihar, Anuj Singh: Host Modulation in Periodontology, Hamburg, Anchor Academic Publishing 2017

Buch-ISBN: 978-3-95489-454-3
PDF-eBook-ISBN: 978-3-95489-954-8
Druck/Herstellung: Anchor Academic Publishing, Hamburg, 2017

Bibliografische Information der Deutschen Nationalbibliothek:
Die Deutsche Nationalbibliothek verzeichnet diese Publikation in der Deutschen Nationalbibliografie; detaillierte bibliografische Daten sind im Internet über http://dnb.d-nb.de abrufbar.

Bibliographical Information of the German National Library:
The German National Library lists this publication in the German National Bibliography. Detailed bibliographic data can be found at: http://dnb.d-nb.de

All rights reserved. This publication may not be reproduced, stored in a retrieval system or transmitted, in any form or by any means, electronic, mechanical, photocopying, recording or otherwise, without the prior permission of the publishers.

Das Werk einschließlich aller seiner Teile ist urheberrechtlich geschützt. Jede Verwertung außerhalb der Grenzen des Urheberrechtsgesetzes ist ohne Zustimmung des Verlages unzulässig und strafbar. Dies gilt insbesondere für Vervielfältigungen, Übersetzungen, Mikroverfilmungen und die Einspeicherung und Bearbeitung in elektronischen Systemen.

Die Wiedergabe von Gebrauchsnamen, Handelsnamen, Warenbezeichnungen usw. in diesem Werk berechtigt auch ohne besondere Kennzeichnung nicht zu der Annahme, dass solche Namen im Sinne der Warenzeichen- und Markenschutz-Gesetzgebung als frei zu betrachten wären und daher von jedermann benutzt werden dürften.

Die Informationen in diesem Werk wurden mit Sorgfalt erarbeitet. Dennoch können Fehler nicht vollständig ausgeschlossen werden und die Diplomica Verlag GmbH, die Autoren oder Übersetzer übernehmen keine juristische Verantwortung oder irgendeine Haftung für evtl. verbliebene fehlerhafte Angaben und deren Folgen.

Alle Rechte vorbehalten

© Anchor Academic Publishing, Imprint der Diplomica Verlag GmbH
Hermannstal 119k, 22119 Hamburg
http://www.diplomica-verlag.de, Hamburg 2017
Printed in Germany

TABLE OF CONTENTS

INTRODUCTION 3

REVIEW OF LITERATURE 6
   A) REVIEW OF LITERATURE ON MODULATION OF
      ARACHIDONIC ACID METABOLITES 6
   B) REVIEW OF LITERATURE ON MODULATION OF HOST
      MATRIX METALLOPROTEINASES 11
   C) REVIEW OF LITERATURE ON MODULATION OF HOST
      CYTOKINES & NITRIC OXIDE SYNTHASE (NOS) ACTIVITY 15
   D) REVIEW OF LITERATURE ON MODULATION OF BONE
      REMODELLING & ENAMEL MATRIX DERIVATIVES AS A
      HOST MODULATION AGENT 17

HOST RESPONSES IN PERIODONTAL DISEASES
– AN OVERVIEW 21
   A) ARACHIDONIC ACID METABOLITES 23
      I) CYCLOOXYGENASE 24
      II) LIPOOXYGENASE 25
      III) ENDOGENOUS ANTI-INFLAMMATORY MEDIATORS
         – LIPOXINS 26
   B) MATRIX METALLOPROTEINASES (MMPS) 30
   C) PRO-INFLAMMATORY CYTOKINES 32
   D) PRODUCTION OF NITRIC OXIDE 35
   E) REGULATION OF BONE REMODELING 37

HOST MODULATION THERAPY 40
   A) MODULATION OF ARACHIDONIC ACID METABOLITES 41
      I) NON STEROIDAL ANTI INFLAMMATORY DRUGS (NSAIDS) ... 42
      II) LIPOXINS (LX) AND ASPIRIN TRIGGERED LIPOXINS (ATL) ... 56
   B) MODULATION OF HOST MATRIX METALLOPROTEINASES 58
      I) CHEMICALLY MODIFIED OR LOW DOSE TETRACYCLINE 60
      II) BISPHOSPHONATE THERAPY 73
      III) SYNTHETIC INHIBITORS OF METALLOPROTEINASES 74

- C) MODULATION OF HOST CYTOKINES 76
- D) MODULATION OF NITRIC OXIDE SYNTHASE (NOS) ACTIVITY . 82
- E) ENAMEL MATRIX PROTEIN AS A HOST MODULATING AGENT 85
- F) MODULATION OF BONE REMODELING 87
  - I) OSTEOPROTEGERIN (OPG) 87
  - II) BISPHOSPHONATES 89

SUMMARY & CONCLUSIONS 104

REFERENCES 106

INTRODUCTION

Periodontitis was believed to be an inevitable consequence of aging & uniformly distributed in population. This age old belief was again supported by another belief that disease severity was directly proportional to plaque levels. But in mid 1990's early insight about complex diseases like periodontitis, led to new conceptual models of pathogenesis.[1] In recent years the role of microorganisms as the principle etiologic factor in periodontal diseases has gained new perspectives. Periodontal disease is a multifactorial & complex disease which is characterized by an up regulated or maladapted immune inflammatory response to bacterial plaque which predisposes to periodontal breakdown. Although periodontal disease is initiated by bacteria colonizing the tooth surface & gingival sulcus, the host response is believed to play an important role in breakdown of connective tissue & bone.[2]

Thus it can be summarized that periodontopathogens are necessary to cause periodontal disease but they are not sufficient to cause the disease. In response to infectious or inflammatory, two distinct yet intricately linked immune response occurs – innate & adaptive. The immune system is essential & the body must be marshal the innate & adaptive responses in order to stave off infection. However, in inflammatory disease the response becomes chronic & tissues do not return to homeostasis.[3] The development of an immune inflammatory response during periodontitis in susceptible individuals results in local production of variety of inflammatory mediators. The development of an immune inflammatory response during periodontitis in susceptible individuals results in local production of variety of inflammatory response during periodontitis in susceptible individuals results in local production of variety of inflammatory mediators. Pro-inflammatory cytokines molecules & cytokine network plays an essential role in pathogenesis of periodontal disease.

Microbial antigens & virulence factors elicit an immediate inflammatory & immune response from the host. The host reacts to microbial insults by producing cytokines, kinins, complement activation & matrix metalloproteinases. Some of these inflammatory mediators participate in periodontal ligament & bone destruction. Constituents of biofilm stimulate host cells to produce a proinflammatory cytokines including IL-1, IL-6 & TNF- which may include connective tissue & alveolar bone resorption.[4] Prostaglandin E2 (PGE2) which may arachidonic acid metabolite play a critical role in regulation of periodontal disease.[5] Moreover, it is consensus that matrix metalloproteinases (MMP's) produced by both infiltrating & resident cells of periodontium plays a role in periodontal disease.[4] Again, it has also been reported that reactive oxygen species (ROS) such as nitric oxide which has been shown to be toxic when present at high levels.[5]

Periodontal treatment, through the ages has focused on the reduction of bacterial infection by mechanical removal of infectious agents i.e (SRP). However, this conventional approach of elimination of infectious agents may not always provide the assurance of a definitive treatment of periodontitis. Thus, this short come has led to use of other sophisticated biological modalities.

Today our knowledge about pathogenesis of periodontal disease has gained new perspectives. This understanding has thus opened new horizon for researchers to explore a novel approach of treatment by means of host response modulation. This treatment concept is aimed at reducing tissue destruction & stabilizing or even regenerate the periodontium by modifying or downregulating the destructive aspects of host response & upregulating protective or regenerative responses. Host modulation therapy offers a potential to move the periodontal treatment to next level.

The various natural inherent defense mechanism have demonstrated to moderate the host response & co-ordinate the resolution of inflammation.

Lipoxins, one such endogenous molecule are liberated during host defense & inflammation have demonstrated as having inflammation resolving properties by stopping signals for polymorphonuclear neutrophils mediated tissue injury.[6] Similarly, it has been shown that imbalance between activated matrix metalloproteinases & their endogenous inhibitors leads to pathological breakdown of extracellular matrix during periodontitis.[4] Moreover, activities of IL-1,TNF-α & interferon-γ are counterimbalanced by production of IL-4, IL-10 & TGF-β.[7] A soluble factor, osteoprotegrin (OPG) binds to RANKL & inhibits the differentiation of osteolcalasts.[8]

Therefore, it appears logical that drug preparations that mimic these endogenous anti-inflammatory mechanisms may prove to be an effective strategy of periodontal treatment. Thus, host modulation therapy (HMT) is designed to block various pathways which are responsible for periodontal disease. These pathways include arachidonic acid metabolites, matrix metalloproteinases, proinflammatory cytokines, production of nitric oxide & regulation bone remodeling. Compared to other treatment approaches host modulation therapy presents as a treatment modality with relatively fewer side effects. Thus host modulation therapy (HMT) may prove to be an effective mode of treating periodontal disease.

Therefore, the aim of this review is to provide comprehensive information & to update about various therapeutic methods to modify the host response as an adjunctive treatment for periodontitis.

REVIEW OF LITERATURE

A) REVIEW OF LITERATURE ON MODULATION OF ARACHIDONIC ACID METABOLITES

1. **Feildman et al (1983)**[74] investigated the effect of non-steroidal anti-inflammatory drugs on the alveolar bone levels in 75 patients with a long term history of aspirin and/or indomethacin therapy. This study concluded that the inhibition of bone loss found in their study could be due to the chronic ingestion of aspirin or aspirin and indomethacin.

2. **Heasman et.al (1989)**[75] investigated the effects of a topical NSAID solution flurbiprofen on the development of experimentally-induced gingivitis in human. The authors concluded that systemic absorption of flurbiprofen reduces the severity of developing inflammatory lesion.

3. **Williams et.al (1989)**[76] examined the effect of the NSAID, flurbiprofen in 56 individuals with radiographic evidence of alveolar bone loss. Subjects were followed a period of 2 years. This study concluded that the NSAID flurbiprofen, as an inhibitor, of cyclooxygenase, can inhibit human alveolar bone loss as measured radiographically.

4. **Reddy et.al (1993)**[77] studied the effect of the non-steroidal anti-inflammatory drug, meclofenamate sodium (Meclomen), as an adjunct to scaling and root planing on the progression of alveolar bone loss associated with rapidly progressive periodontitis (RPP). Based on the observations obtained from this study, the authors concluded that meclofenamate sodium

may have a potential role in treatment regimens for patients with rapidly progressive periodontitis.

5. **Heasman et.al (1993)**[78] examined the effects of a potent cyclooxygenase inhibitor, flurbiprofen, on both clinical parameters and on release of PGE_2, TxB_2 and LTB_4 during the development of inflammation using the experimental gingivitis model in 21 humans. The authors reported that flurbiprofen controls gingival inflammation at both preventive and therapeutic levels in the experimental gingivitis model and suggested that this effect could be associated with an inhibition in the production of cyclooxygenase metabolites that indirectly affects GCF- LTB_4 levels.

6. **Heasman et.al (1994)**[79] conducted a study which was aimed at investigating the effect of a systemic flurbiprofen preparation (100 mg daily) on the resolution of experimental gingivitis in 47 human volunteers. The authors concluded that the flurbiprofen has a beneficial effect by increasing the rate of resolution of inflammation.

7. **Jeffcoat et al (1995)**[80] assessed the efficacy of a topical NSAID rinse, containing ketorolac tromethamine as the active agent. 55 adult periodontitis patients were studied in this 6-month study. Systemic flurbiprofen was used as a positive control. Standardized radiographs were taken at baseline, at 3 and at 6 months by digital subtraction radiography. It was concluded that ketorolac rinse preserved more alveolar bone than systemic flurbiprofen and that ketorolac rinse may be beneficial in the treatment of adult periodontitis.

8. **Preshaw et.al (1998)**[81] investigated the effects of topical ketorolac tromethamine mouthrinse (0.1%) on gingival crevicular fluid (GCF)

prostaglandin E_2 (PGE_2) concentrations. This study concluded that ketorolac mouth rinse controlled the elevation of GCF PGE2 compared to placebo, but did not actually reduced GCF PGE2 concentrations.

9. **Bichara et.al (1999)**[82] studied the effect of a one week course of postsurgical naproxen (500mg, twice daily for one week) on the osseous healing in intrabony defects treated with polylactide bioabsorbable membranes. The observations obtained form the study stated that, an administration of postsurgical naproxen did not produce superior defect fill compared to that obtained with polylactide bioabsorbable membranes alone.

10. **Pouliot et.al (1999)**[83] investigated the impact of metabolically stable LX and ATL analogues on TNF-α induced neutrophil response. The authors concluded that both LXA4 and ATL are regulators of TNF α -directed neutrophil actions and stimulate IL-4 to play an important role in preventing periodontal disease.

11. **Bezerra M. (2000)**[84] compared the effect of selective COX-2 inhibitors – meloxicam and indomethacin on alveolar bone loss (ABL) in an experimental periodontitis model in rats. The authors suggested that both indomethacin and meloxicam prevented ABL and reduced inflammatory changes through COX inhibition. They also observed that meloxicam displays similar efficacy and less gastric damage than indomethacin.

12. **Paquette et.al (2000)**[85] evaluated the pharmacodynamic effects of the NSAID, ketoprofen on gingival crevicular fluid (GCF) prostanoids. The authors concluded that both topical and systemic ketoprofen therapies pharmacodynamically reduce GCF PGE_2 levels in adult periodontitis subjects resulting in inhibition of disease progression.

13. **Holzhausen et.al (2002)**[86] studied the effect of a selective cyclooxygenase-2 inhibitor (celecoxib) on alveolar bone resorption in experimentally induced periodontal disease in rats. It was concluded that the systemic therapy with the celecoxib could modify the progression of experimentally induced periodontitis in rats.

14. **Vardar et.al (2003)**[87] compared the effects of selective cyclooxygenase (COX)-2 inhibitor (nimesulide) and non-selective COX-1/COX-2 inhibitor (naproxen) as an adjunct to non-surgical (SRP) periodontal therapy in chronic periodontitis patients on the gingival tissue levels of prostaglandin PGE_2 and $PGF_{2\alpha}$. The authors concluded that nimesulide may have additional inhibitory effects on gingival tissue $PGF_{2\alpha}$ levels in the first week following non-surgical periodontal treatment. However, it has an insignificant effect on reducing PGE_2 levels in gingival tissue.

15. *Serhan et.al (2003)*[88] concluded LXs can be targets for novel approaches to diseases, e.g., periodontitis and arthritis, where inflammation and bone destruction are features.

16. **Gurgel et.al (2004)**[89] conducted a study which stated that selective cyclooxygenase-2 inhibitors may reduce bone loss associated with experimental periodontitis and that there is no remaining effect after its withdrawal.

17. **Sekino et.al (2005)**[90] conducted a study on eleven subjects to evaluate the effect of systemic administration of ibuprofen on gingivitis and de novo plaque formation. The authors concluded that ibuprofen administered via the systemic route has an effect on gingivitis but not on de novo plaque formation.

18. Kurtis et.al (2007)[91] investigated the effect of systemic flurbiprofen administration as an adjunct to SRP in smoker and non-smoker patients with chronic periodontitis. therapy, a more statistically significant reduction was observed in group 3. The authors concluded that better results were found in smokers as compared to non smokers.

19. C. Alec Yen et al (2008)[92] tested the efficacy of celecoxib (COX-2 inhibitor) in conjunction with scaling and root planing (SRP) in subjects with chronic periodontitis (CP). This study concluded that celecoxib can be an effective adjunctive treatment to SRP to reduce progressive attachment loss in subjects with CP.

20. Thais M. Oliveira et al (2008)[93] evaluated the effect of a preferential cyclooxygenase (COX)-2 inhibitor meloxicam on VEGF expression and alveolar bone loss in experimentally induced periodontitis. The data of this study suggested that systemic therapy with meloxicam can modify the progression of experimentally induced periodontitis in rats by reducing VEGF expression and alveolar bone loss.

B) REVIEW OF LITERATURE ON MODULATION OF HOST MATRIX METALLOPROTEINASES

1. **Golub et.al. (1995)**[94] evaluated the effect of low-dose doxycycline on host-derived collagenase activity in gingival tissues of adult periodontitis patient. They concluded that the pathologically-elevated tissue-degrading activities can be directly inhibited by pharmacologic levels of doxycyline.

2. **Crout et.al (1996)**[95] investigated the clinical results of a "cyclical" 6-month regimen of low dose doxycyline and its effect on GCF collagenase activity in adult periodontitis patients. The authors concluded that low dose doxycycline inhibits tissue destruction in the absence of either antimicrobial or significant anti-inflammatory efficacy; and that long-term low dose doxycycline could be a useful adjunct to instrumentation therapy in the management of the adult periodontitis patient.

3. **Veronica and Bisada (1998)**[96] compared the efficacy of the combined systemic use of doxycycline and a non-steroidal anti-inflammatory drug (ibuprofen),as an adjunctive treatment to scaling and root planing for adult periodontitis. . The authors concluded that systemic doxycycline alone or in combination with ibuprofen results in a statistically significant yet modest clinical improvement in patients with moderate adult periodontitis.

4. **Caton et.al (2000)**[97] conducted a study which assessed the efficacy of subantimicrobial dose doxycycline in conjunction with scaling and root planing (SRP) over a 9 month period in patients with adult periodontitis. They concluded that the use of SDD 20 mg twice daily augment the attachment gains achieved with SRP, with statistically significant

improvements in CAL and PD relative to placebo after only 3 months of use and further improvements were evident after 6 months of SDD treatment.

5. **H. Nakaya et al (2000)**[98] investigated the regulatory effects of a bisphosphonate, tiludronate, on MMP levels and activity in human periodontal cells. This study demonstrated an inhibitory effect of tiludronate on the activity of both MMP-1 and MMP-3.

6. **Golub et.al (2001)**[99] carried out a study to determine appropriate dosage of administration regimens using subantimicrobial dose doxycycline (SDD) as an adjunctive therapy in patients with adult periodontitis. This study concluded that the administration of 20 mg of twice daily over an extended period can reduce pathologic elevations in GCF collagenase activity and improve attachment level measurements in patients with periodontitis and that the improvement in parameters occurred without any apparent side effects.

7. **Ramamurthy et.al (2002)**[100] tested the efficacy of doxycycline and 5 different chemically modified tetracyclines (CMTs) to prevent matrix metalloproteinase (MMP)-dependent periodontal tissue breakdown in an animal model of periodontitis. The authors concluded that MMP-mediated bone loss in this model can be prevented by inhibition of MMPs using CMTs.

8. **Novak et.al (2002)**[101] studied the use of adjunctive host modulation therapy in form of subantimicrobial doxycycline (SDD) for treating severe, generalized periodontitis. The authors concluded that SDD as an adjunctive treatment provides clinically and statistically significant benefits in the reduction of deep pockets in patients with severe, generalized periodontitis.

9. **Emingil et.al (2004)**[102] studied the impact of Low-dose doxycycline (LDD) in combination with non-surgical periodontal therapy on gingival crevicular fluid (GCF) matrix metalloproteinase-8 (MMP-8) levels as well as on clinical parameters over a 12-month period in patients with chronic periodontitis. The authors concluded that adjunctive low-dose doxycycline therapy in combination with scaling and root planing (SRP) reduces GCF MMP-8 levels and improves clinical parameters in patients with chronic periodontitis. They also suggested that greatest benefit of adjunctive low-dose doxycycline therapy on clinical parameters could occur about 9 months after therapy.

10. **Gapski et.al (2004)**[103] evaluated the efficacy of access flap surgery with and without supplemental SDD for 6 months among individuals (n=24) previously unresponsive to scaling and root planing. They noted that SDD lead to statistically significant greater probing depth reduction at sites initially more then 6 mm deep .SDD administration also resulted in a greater reduction of levels of ICTP (a carboxyterminal fragment of type 1 collagen), which is a marker for bone resorption.

11. **Gurkan et.al, (2005)**[104] stated that combination of SDD with non-surgical therapy improves clinical parameters of periodontal disease and increases GCF TGF-beta1 levels together with a decrease in prevalence.

12. **Preshaw et.al (2005)**[105] concluded that adjunctive SDD enhances therapeutic outcomes compared with SRP alone, resulting in clinical benefit in both smokers and non-smokers with chronic periodontitis.

13. **Buduneli et.al (2007)**[106] suggested that the combined administration of doxycycline and alendronate may provide beneficial effects in periodontal

treatment. They also suggested that alendronate and/or doxycycline may inhibit MMP-8 expression significantly and individual administration of alendronate and doxycycline results in significant increase in TIMP-1 expression in gingiva.

14. **G. Emingil (2008)**[107] examined the effectiveness of a 3-month regimen of subantimicrobial dose doxycycline (SDD) in combination with SRP compared to SRP alone on levels of gingival crevicular fluid (GCF) extracellular matrix metalloproteinase inducer (EMMPRIN) in patients with chronic periodontitis. The authors concluded that SDD therapy in combination with scaling and root planing reduced GCF EMMPRIN levels and improved clinical periodontal parameters in subjects with chronic periodontitis.

15. **Golub. M et al (2008)**[108] tested the hypothesis of subantimicrobial-dose doxycycline modulating gingival crevicular fluid biomarkers of periodontitis in postmenopausal (PM) osteopenic women. The observations of the study support the therapeutic potential of long-term SDD therapy to reduce periodontal collagen breakdown and alveolar bone resorption in PM women

C) REVIEW OF LITERATURE ON MODULATION OF HOST CYTOKINES & NITRIC OXIDE SYNTHASE (NOS) ACTIVITY

1. **Assuma et al. (1998)**[109] investigated the effects of function-blocking soluble receptors to IL-1 and TNF in ligature-induced experimental periodontitis in animal model. The results indicated that injection of soluble receptors to IL-1 and TNF inhibited by approximately 80% the recruitment of inflammatory cells in close proximity to bone and the amount of bone loss was reduced by 60%.

2. **Graves et.al (1998)**[110] studied the effect of topical application of soluble receptors to IL-1 and TNF on progression of inflammatory cells towards alveolar bone in primate model of experimental periodontitis. The authors concluded that local injection of soluble receptors to IL-1 and TNF inhibited osteoclast formation and progression of inflammatory cell infiltration towards alveolar bone.

3. **Lohinai et.al, (1998)**[111] investigated the potential protective effect of mercaptoethylguanidine (MEG) on the bone loss associated with periodontitis in ligature induced periodontitis in rats. The results of the study showed that ligature-induced periodontitis showed increase in local NO production and that MEG treatment protects against the associated extravasation and bone destruction.

4. **Martuscelli et al. (2000)**[112] studied the effects of recombinant human IL-11 (rhIL-11) by subcutaneous administration to prevent progression of attachment loss and radiographic bone loss in a ligature induced periodontitis in beagle dog model. The authors concluded that the

subcutaneous injections of rhIL-11 can inhibit the progression of attachment loss and radiographic bone loss in experimental periodontitis model.

5. **Delima (2001)**[113] studied effect of topical application of soluble receptors to IL-1 and TNF on preventing loss of connective tissue attachment, thereby preventing progression of periodontitis in a primate model of experimental periodontitis. The authors concluded that the loss of connective tissue attachment and progression of periodontal disease can be retarded by antagonists to specific host mediators such as IL-1 and TNF.

6. **Oates et.al (2002)**[114] assessed clinical, radiographic, and biochemical markers as diagnostic indicators of disease activity by comparing ligature-induced bone loss in the presence or absence of IL-1/TNF-α antagonist inhibition of bone loss in a primate model. The use of the blockers significantly reduced the levels of radiographic bone loss by approximately 50%. No significant effect on GI, and GCF amounts were observed.

7. **Lohinai et al. (2003)**[115] investigated the role of the activation of nuclear poly (ADP-ribose) polymerase (PARP) enzyme, a mediator of downstream nitric oxide toxicity, in a ligature-induced-periodontitis model in rats and mice. Thus, PARP activation contributes to the development of periodontal injury. Inhibition of PARP may represent a novel host response modulatory approach for the therapy of periodontitis.

D) REVIEW OF LITERATURE ON MODULATION OF BONE REMODELLING & ENAMEL MATRIX DERIVATIVES AS A HOST MODULATION AGENT

1. **Brunsvold et.al (1992)**[116] determined the effect of a bisphosphonate compound on the development of periodontitis using the non-human primate model. The authors concluded that alendronate, a bisphosphonate, significantly inhibited bone density loss in periodontitis without significantly affecting the plaque index, gingival index or probing depth measurements.

2. **Weinreb et.al (1994)**[117] tested the efficacy of alendronate, a bisphosphonate, in reducing alveolar bone loss caused by experimental periodontitis in monkeys. The authors concluded that alendronate could reduce the loss of alveolar bone support associated with periodontitis.

3. **Yaffe et.al (1995)**[118] tested the ability of amino hydroxybutylidene bisphosphonate (AB) to suppress alveolar bone loss during the initial phase of regional accelerated phenomenon following mucoperiosteal flap surgery. This study showed that administration of 0.5 mg/kg body weight of AB demonstrated marked reduction of bone resorption. The authors suggested prescribing the AB for patients before periodontal or implant surgery, and following surgery is beneficial to prevent or minimize bone resorption.

4. **Shoji et.al (1995)**[119] examined the effect of systemic administration of a bisphosphonate, risedronate, on alveolar bone loss in experimental periodontitis. The authors concluded that administration of risedronate could be effective in preventing bone resorption in periodontitis.

5. **Yaffe et.al (1997)**[120] evaluated the effect of local delivery of the amino bisphosphonate on bone resorption as an adjuvant to mucoperiosteal flaps. The authors concluded that local application of amino bisphosphonate could be used as an adjunct in therapy for reducing bone resorption following surgery.

6. **Ouchi (1998)**[121] examined the efficacy of YM 175 (disodium cycloheptylaminomethylenediphosphonate monohydrate) in reducing alveolar bone loss caused by experimental periodontitis in beagle dogs. The authors concluded that YM 175 could prevent alveolar bone loss by reducing the alveolar bone turnover in dogs with periodontitis.

7. **Binderman et.al (2000)**[122] investigated the effectiveness of different concentrations of alendronate delivery at the surgical site during the time of surgery, in reducing alveolar bone loss. The authors concluded that topical delivery of alendronate at the time of surgery reduces bone loss in periodontal procedures.

8. **Alencar et.al (2002)**[123] studied the effects of administrating disodium chlodronate to rats in an experimental periodontitis model. The authors concluded that disodium chlodronate has both bone sparing and anti-inflammatory activity when administered as a pretreatment or in an ongoing process.

9. **Kaynak et.al (2003)**[124] examined histopathologically the effect of systemic administration of aminobisphosphonate (alendronate) on alveolar bone resorption following mucoperiosteal flap surgery in rats. The observations of this study showed that the systemic administration of 0.5 mg/kg

alendronate could be effective in preventing alveolar bone loss and in modulating tissue factors.

10. **Takaishi Y et.al (2003)**[125] used intermittent cyclical **etidronate** for 4-5 years in addition to ordinary dental therapy in four women with periodontitis. This study showed that there was an increase in alveolar bone density which was associated with the clinical benefits of etidronate in the treatment of periodontitis.

11. **Rocha et.al (2004)**[126] investigated the effect of oral alendronate treatment on radiological and clinical measurements of periodontal disease in postmenopausal women without hormone replacement therapy. The authors concluded that alendronate may be useful in treating periodontal disease in postmenopausal women.

12. **Mohamed H. Parkar et al (2004)**[127] conducted a study to explore the selective effects of EMD on the activities of 268 cytokine, growth factor, and receptor genes in PDL. The present study has shown that EMD downregulates the expression of genes involved in the early inflammatory phases of wound healing while simultaneously upregulating genes encoding growth and repair-promoting molecules. This may partly explain the apparent efficacy of EMD application in periodontal regeneration.

13. **Lane et.al (2005)**[128] carried out a study to determine the effect of 1 year bisphosphonate therapy in conjunction with conventional non-surgical treatment in patients with moderate to severe chronic periodontitis. The authors concluded that bisphosphonate treatment may be an appropriate adjunctive treatment to preserve periodontal bone mass and can lead to improved clinical outcome of non-surgical periodontal therapy.

14. **Juan A. Goya et al (2006)[129] studied the** effect of topical administration of monosodium olpadronate (OPD) on experimental periodontitis (EP) in rats. The authors concluded that monosodium olpadronate (OPD) was found to inhibit bone loss and to cause marked morphologic changes in osteoclasts. Thus the drug effectively prevented bone loss caused by periodontitis.

15. **Gabriela Giro et al (2007)[130] conducted a** study which investigated the influence of estrogen deficiency and its treatment with estrogen and alendronate on the removal torque of osseointegrated titanium implants. According to this study, estrogen deficiency was observed to have a negative influence on the removal torque of osseointegrated implants, whereas treatment with alendronate increased the torque needed to remove the implants.

16. **Palmo L et al (2007)[131]** in a review of bisphosphonate therapy stated that alveolar bone loss in periodontitis and skeletal bone loss share common mechanisms. Periodontal therapy using bisphosphonates to modulate host response to bacterial insult may develop into a potential strategy in populations in which periodontal therapy is not convenient.

17. **Qiming Jin et al (2007)[132]** evaluated the effect of osteoprotegrin (OPG) on RANKL inhibition & its effects on alveolar bone resorption. The authors concluded that systemic delivery of OPG-Fc inhibits alveolar bone resorption in experimental periodontitis.

18. **Sunao Sato et al (2008)[133]** conducted a study which was aimed at evaluating the influence of EMD on inflammatory-associated markers using an in vitro monocyte assay. This study concluded that that EMD modulates two inflammation-associated factors, TNF-α and PGE_2, in monocytes.

HOST RESPONSES IN PERIODONTAL DISEASES – AN OVERVIEW

It is now established & supported by enormous data that plaque biofilm and associated host response are involved in the pathogenesis of periodontal disease. The microbial challenge stimulates host responses which result in disease limited to the gingiva (i.e gingivitis) or initiation of periodontitis. Host response also involves protective aspects which include recruitment of neutrophils, production of protective antibodies, and possibly the release of anti-inflammatory cytokines including transforming growth factor-ß (TGF- ß), interleukin-4 (IL-4), IL-10, and IL-11 (Page & Kornman 1997).[9] Perpetuation of the host response due to persistent bacterial challenge disrupts homeostatic mechanisms and results in recruitment of neutrophils, macrophages, and release of mediators including pro-inflammatory cytokines, matrix metalloproteinases, arachidonic acid metabolites, reactive oxygen species, as well as release of mediators for osteoclastic bone resorption.

Host cells are stimulated by constituents of the biofilm to produce pro-inflammatory cytokines including IL-1β, IL-6 and tumor necrosis factor-α (TNF-α), which may induce connective tissue and alveolar bone destruction.[10] These cytokines have been observed in diseased periodontal tissues and gingival crevicular fluid (GCF). The catabolic activities to these cytokines are known to control by endogenous inhibitors that include IL-1, and TNF receptor antagonists.[10] Other hypothesis regarding periodontal disease pathogenesis is that host cells stimulated directly or indirectly by components of the plaque biofilm secrete the matrix metalloproteinases. Matrix metalloproteinases are released by a variety of infiltrating cells[11] (i.e neutrophils and macrophages) and resident cells[12] (i.e by fibroblasts, epithelial cells, osteoblast and osteoclast) found in the periodontium. These matrix metalloproteinases are primarily responsible for connective tissue destruction.

Moreover, another pathway involved in periodontal disease pathogenesis is the synthesis and release of prostaglandins and other arachidonic acid metabolites within periodontal tissues. Both bacterial and host factors initiate tissue damage. This damage allows phospholipids in plasma membranes of cells to become available for action by phospholipase and thereby results in production of free arachidonic acid. Arachidonic acid can be metabolized via cyclooxygenase (CO) or lipoxygenase (LO) pathways. The final products of the CO pathway include prostaglandins, prostacyclins, and thromboxanes, whereas the end results of the LO pathway include leukotrienes (LTs) and other hydroxyeicosatetraenoic acids. Elevated levels of prostaglandins and other arachidonic acid metabolites have been reported[13] in GCF and periodontal tissues in patients exhibiting gingivitis, periodontitis. Host cells also releases mediators including reactive oxygen species[14] which are antagonist to plaque biofilms, but which in excess may initiate inflammation. For example, nitric oxide is a free radical involved in host defense that can be toxic when present at high levels and it has been implicated in a variety of inflammatory conditions.[15] Recent developments in the area of mediators of osteoclastic differentiation have expanded our knowledge of the process of bone resorption.[16]

The components of immune inflammatory responses of periodontal disease pathogenesis are discussed here under following headings: arachidonic acid metabolites, matrix metalloproteinases, pro-inflammatory cytokines, production of nitric oxide, and regulation of bone remodeling.

A) ARACHIDONIC ACID METABOLITES

Arachidonic acid is a 20 carbon essential fatty acid (eicosanoid) which is normally present in mammalian cells in an esterified form within membrane phospholipids and is liberated from it by the action of phospholipase enzyme. Free arachidonic acid is metabolized via either the cyclooxygenase (CO) or lipoxygenase (LO) pathways. The cyclooxygenase pathway ultimately results in the synthesis of the prostaglandins, thromboxanes, and prostacyclins. The lipoxygenase pathway leads to the hydroxyeicosatetraenoic acids (HETES) and the leukotrienes (LTs). In addition, a series of oxygenated arachidonic acid derivatives called lipoxins are formed by interactions between individual LO.

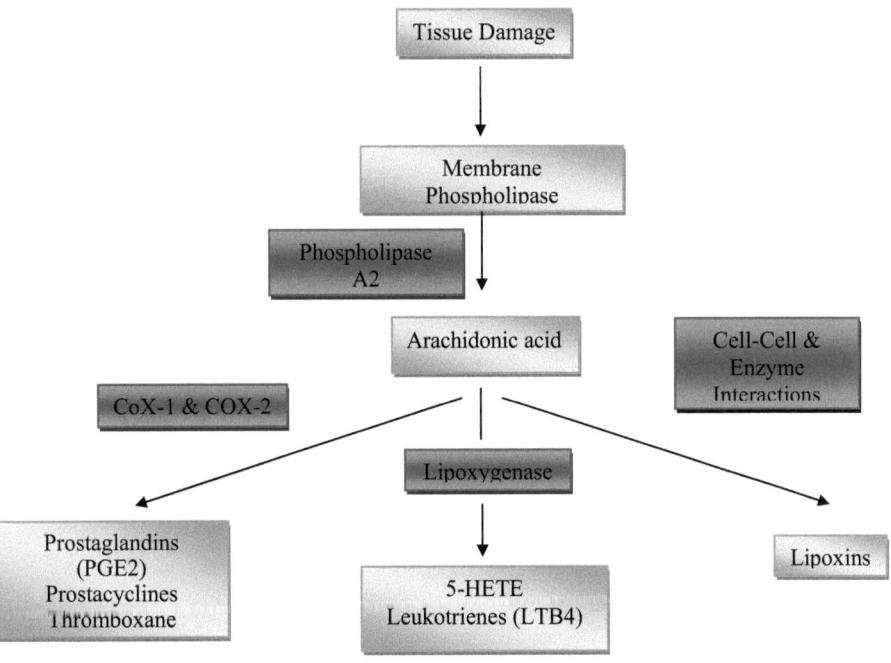

Fig.1

I) Cyclooxygenase

There are two isoforms of the enzyme COX which have been identified.[17] COX-1 is a constitutive enzyme expressed in most cells and tissues, and appears to represent an essential component of tissue homeostasis. In contrast, COX-2 represents an inducible isoform localized primarily in inflamed tissues [18] and is upregulated by IL-1β, TNF-α, bacteria and lipopolysaccharide (LPS).[19] Cells stimulated with cytokines such as IL-1β or LPS are able to rapidly synthesize COX-2 from pre-existing mRNA and translate new COX-2 transcripts, leading to a prolonged COX-2 release without inducing COX-1 biosynthesis.

The other arachidonic acid metabolites such as prostacyclin and LT appeared to be actively involved in bone resorption. Prostacyclin (PGI_2) is an endothelial cell product capable of preventing platelet aggregation and platelet adhesion to vessel walls.[20] Findings from tissue culture experiments demonstrated that PGI_2 stimulated bone resorption.[21]

Prostagladin E_2

Prostaglandin E_2 has diverse proinflammatory and immunomodulatory effects. PGE_2 induces vasodilation and increased capillary permeability which elicit clinical signs of redness and edema. PGE_2 also enhances inflammatory cell infiltration, not as a chemoattractant, but by abrogating the chemotactic migration and egress of neutrophils and other inflammatory cells which have been recruited to the site of infection by chemoattractants such as LTB4. At the site of infection PGE_2 can down-regulate or stabilize newly-recruited neutrophils to prevent premature degranulation and oxidative burst prior to bacterial confrontation. PGE_2 is a potent inducer of MMP secretion by monocytes and fibroblasts to trigger connective tissue destruction.[22] Osteoclastic bone resorption is also triggered by PGE_2. PGE_2 interacts synergistically with IL-1 and TNF □ to enhance the effects of these molecules.

PGE_2 is easily detected in the GCF and increases 2- to 3-fold in gingivitis and periodontitis, relative to health, and increases another 5- to 6-fold during periods of active disease progression, as determined by longitudinal attachment loss.[23]

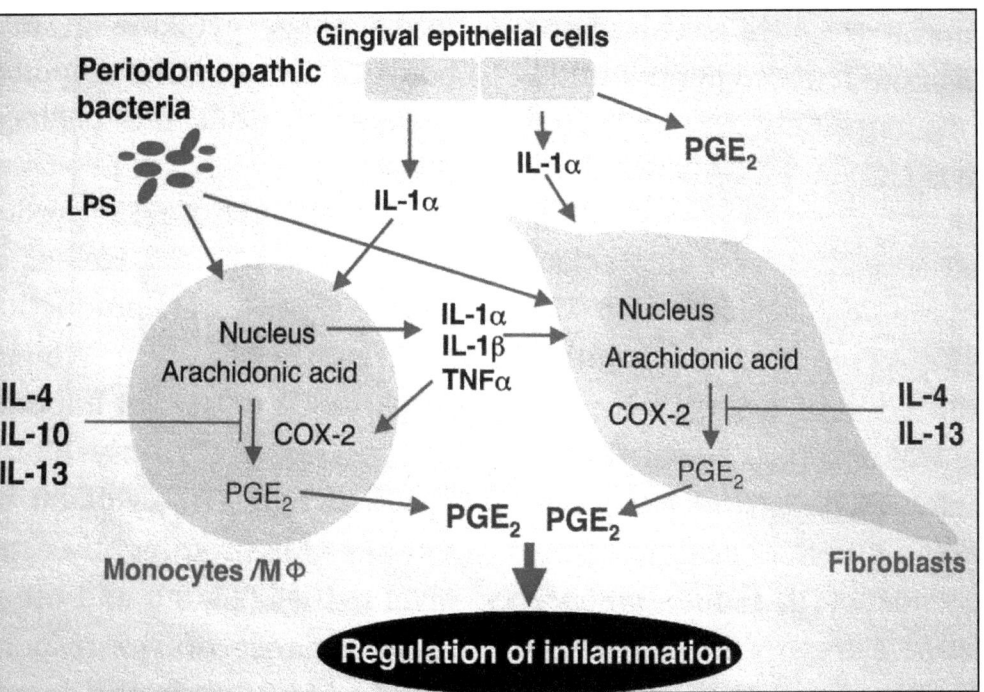

Fig.2. Hypothetical regulatory mechanism of cyclo-oxygenase-2 (COX-2) expression & PGE2 production through cell-cell interaction in periodontal lesions.

II) Lipooxygenase

Arachidonic acid is enzymatically oxidized by the action of lipooxygenase to form leukotrienes (LTs) and other monohydroxy eicosatetraenoic acids. Three different lipooxygenases insert oxygen into the 5, 12 and 15 positions of arachidonic acid, giving rise to hydroperoxidases of eicosatetraenoic acids (HETE). The lipoxygenases 5-LO, 12-LO, and 15-LO are found in neutrophils, platelets, and endothelial/ epithelial cells, respectively, and their products are also named accordingly (5-HETE, 12-HETE, and 15-HETE).[24] The leukotrienes are generated through the lipoxygenase (LO) pathway (Lee and Austen, 1986).[25] The first leukotriene that is formed is LTA4, which in turn is metabolized into either LTB4 or LTC4. Through this process, a peptide glutathione is added to LTC4. LTC4 is converted into LTD4 and LTE4 by the removal of glutamate and glycine.

LTB4 is a product of the lipoxygenase pathway and is the principal product of arachidonic acid metabolism in stimulated human neutrophils.[26] This potent chemotactic mediator plays a central role in the recruitment of PMNs and monocytes to sites of developing gingival inflammation. LTB4 enhances bacterial opsonization.[27] LTB4 also triggers neutrophil degranulation with the release of lysosomal enzymes, elastase, collagenase, and elaboration of superoxide and prostaglandin E_2.[27] Thus, LTB4 release from neutrophils serves to recruit and activate other neutrophils to amplify the inflammatory response.

Meghji S (1988)[29] showed that both leukotrienes and HETEs are potent stimulators of bone resorption and play an important role in the localized bone loss associated with inflammatory lesions. Further evidence in support of the lipoxygenase pathway contributing to bone resorption was found in a study by Gallwitz et al (1993).[30].

III) Endogenous anti-Inflammatory mediators – Lipoxins

Endogenous lipid-derived mediators have been demonstrated to moderate the host response and coordinate the resolution of inflammation.[31] Recently, several novel lipid mediators have been described as potential anti-inflammatory molecules, illustrating the importance of endogenous generation of lipid mediators with anti-inflammatory properties. An important example of lipid mediators with inflammation-resolving properties is the lipoxins (LX). Lipoxins are a series of oxygenated arachidonic acid derivatives formed by interaction between individual LO and appear to function as endogenous anti-inflammatory mediators. Lipoxins contain a trihydroxytetraene group and are members of the eicosanoid family that are produced within the vascular lumen, primarily *via* platelet-leukocyte transcellular biosynthesis.[32]

Lipoxins can be generated by several different pathways. In general, cell-cell interactions result in the generation of lipoxins, while single cells also can produce lipoxins.[33] Lipoxin generation is a very rapid process that is activated by inflammation, atherosclerosis, and thrombosis.[34]

(a) 15-lipoxygenase-initiated pathway

Biosynthesis of lipoxin was first demonstrated in 1984 (Serhan *et al.*, 1984).[35] It was shown that insertion of molecular oxygen into the 15-carbon (C15) position of arachidonic acid is essential for lipoxin production. In addition, it was also reported that lipoxin generation through this pathway required the action of 15-LO. Once oxygenated at the C15 position, arachidonic acid is converted into 15-hydroperoxyeicosatetraenoic acid (15- HPETE), which is a substrate for 5-LO in leukocytes.[36] This molecule is rapidly converted by hydrolases to either lipoxin A4 (LXA4) and/or lipoxin B4 (LXB4). LXA4 and LXB4 are vasoactive molecules, primarily vasodilatory *in vivo*, and regulate leukocyte functions.[37]

(b) 5-lipoxygenase-initiated pathway

The second route for LX biosynthesis occurs with the interaction of human neutrophils with platelets in the blood vessels. In this model, cell-to-cell interaction involves 5-LO in neutrophils and 12-LO in platelets for the insertion of molecular oxygen into arachidonic acid.[38] Under resting conditions, the majority of neutrophil-generated LTA4 by the 5-LO pathway is released into the extracellular environment.[38] When platelets adhere to neutrophils, LTA4 is converted either to LXB4 or LXA4 by 12LO.

(c) Aspirin-triggered lipoxins
Aspirin may also play an important role in the generation of lipoxins.[39] In this transcellular biosynthetic scheme, cyclooxygenase-2 (COX-2) switches its catalytic activity in the presence of aspirin, generating 15R-HETE instead of prostaglandins. Thus, aspirin inhibits prostaglandin biosynthesis by both COX-1 and COX-2.[40] COX-2, when acetylated by aspirin in endothelial or epithelial cells, is enzymatically active and converts arachidonic acid to 15R-HETE, which is released and transformed through transcellular routes to form 15-epi-lipoxins by leukocytes. 15-epi- LXA4 is more potent than native LXA4 in inhibiting Aspirin-triggered lipoxins (ATL) can serve as potential endogenous anti-inflammatory signals or mediators are some of aspirin's beneficial actions. 15-epi-LXA4 and LXA4 analogs inhibit interleukin-1b (IL-lb), tumor necrosis factor-a (TNF-a), and IL-8 expression while stimulating IL-4 release *in vivo*.[41]

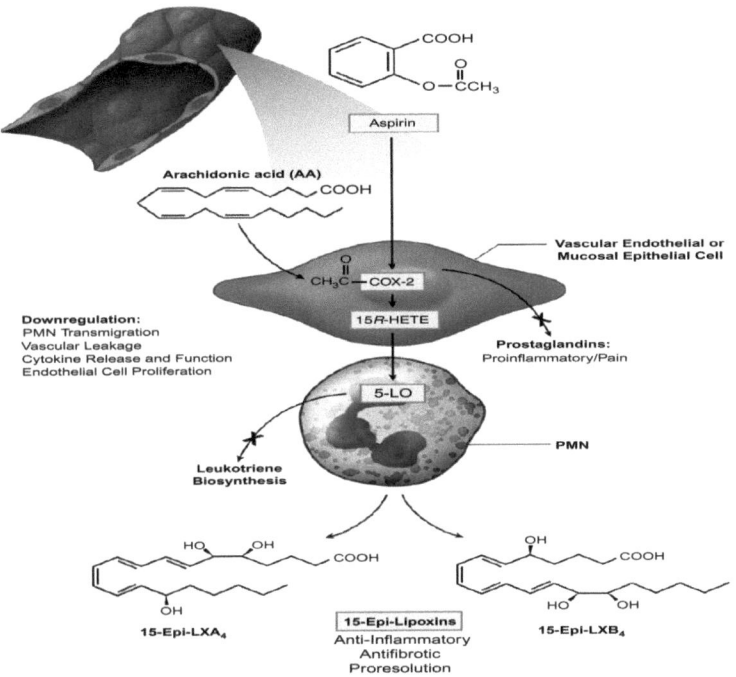

Fig.3. Biosynthesis of ATLs. Under this scenario, acetylated COX-2 does not produce prostaglandin (proinflammatory) intermediates but remains enzymatically active to produce 15R-HETE from AA that is converted by PMN leukocytes to 15-epi-lipoxins. In addition, there is inhibition of leukotrienes (proinflammatory) that are normally initially generated via the 5-LO pathway.

Lipoxins and periodontal diseases

Recently, it was demonstrated that lipoxins are produced by peripheral blood neutrophils from patients diagnosed with aggressive periodontitis. In addition, GCF samples from localized aggressive periodontitis (LAP) patients were examined and found to contain prostaglandin PGE_2, 5-LO-derived products - LTB4, and LXA4. In a mouse model, it was shown that the administration of metabolically stable analogues of lipoxin and of aspirin-triggered lipoxin potently blocked P. gingivalis elicited neutrophil infiltration and lowered PGE2 levels within exudates without allowing infection to spread. Moreover, they provide strong support for the notion that lipoxin can have a protective role in periodontitis, limiting further neutrophil recruitment and neutrophil-mediated tissue injury that can lead to loss of inflammatory barriers that prevent tissue invasion by oral microbial pathogens (Pouliot *et al.*, 2000).[42] These results support the concept that lipoxins may be involved in the regulation of local acute inflammatory response in periodontal disease.

B) <u>MATRIX METALLOPROTEINASES (MMPs)</u>

The matrix metalloproteinases are an important family of zinc - and calcium-dependent endopeptidases secreted or released by a variety of host cells such as polymorphonuclear leukocytes, macrophages, fibroblasts, bone, epithelial and endothelial. Both secreted and membrane-bound MMPs catalyse the breakdown of proteins located either on the cell plasma membrane or within the extracellular matrix, including collagen, gelatin, proteoglycans core protein, fibronectin, laminin and elastin.[43]

Regulation of MMP activity involves specific, endogenous tissue inhibitors of MMPs (TIMPs) and γ macroglobulins, which form complexes with active MMPs, and in some cases with latent MMP precursors.[44] It has been shown that an imbalance between activated matrix metalloproteinases and their host-derived endogenous inhibitors leads to pathological breakdown of the extracellular matrix during periodontitis and numerous other diseases.[45]

In healthy tissues, collagen turnover is a controlled intracellular event that is mediated extracellularly by fibroblast derived collagenase (MMP-1) and intracellularly by a variety of lysosomal acid-dependent enzymes. In inflamed periodontal tissues, the balance between MMPs and TIMPs is disrupted as a result of pathological alterations in the types and quantities of MMPs present. This leads to excessive breakdown of extracellular collagen and inappropriate destruction of periodontal tissues. MMP expression alters in inflamed tissues relative to non-inflamed tissues because each of the major cell types in the periodontium expresses, when appropriately stimulated, a unique combination of MMPs.[46] Transcription of MMP genes is upregulated by pro-inflammatory mediators known to be important in periodontal disease progression, including interleukin- 1α and β (IL-1α and β) and tumor necrosis factor- α (TNF- α).[47]

The evidence for the role of matrix metalloproteinases in periodontal destruction is strong and has been supported over many years by a number of findings, including the production of elevated levels of collagenase by diseased gingival tissues in culture.[48] Inflammatory cells such as neutrophils and macrophages produce matrix metalloproteinases, with neutrophils being the major source of collagenase and gelatinase in inflammatory diseases such as periodontitis.[49] It has been identified that the predominant MMPs (in particular MMP-8 and MMP-9) in GCF in periodontitis patients derive from PMNs (Golub et al. 1998b).[50] These MMPs are particularly effective in degrading type-1 collagen, which is the predominant collagen type in gingiva and PDL.[51] Markedly increased expression of MMP-13 has been seen in gingival sections of subjects with chronic periodontitis.[52] Thus, the predominant MMPs in inflamed gingival and periodontal tissues are PMN-type MMPs (MMP-8 and MMP-9) and bone-derived MMP-13, rather than fibroblast-type MMP (MMP-1).[53] Levels of PMN-type MMPs & MMP-13 have been shown to increase with increasing periodontal disease severity and decrease following therapy.[54] Matrix metalloproteinase-9 (gelatinase-B) were also found to be secreted by human osteoclasts *in vitro*.[55]

In periodontal diseases, matrix metalloproteinases play key roles in the degradation of the extracellular matrix, basement membrane and protective serpins as well as in modifying the action of cytokine and activation of osteoclasts., The extracellular matrix not only consists of collagen fibrils but also their associated proteoglycans and fibronectin, which must be removed first in order for the collagenase to have access to the collagen substrate. Matrix metalloproteinase-3 (stromelysin) is effective at degrading proteoglycans and fibronectin.

Endogenous Matrix metalloproteinase inhibitors

Matrix metalloproteinases secreted from various host cells catalyze the breakdown of proteins located either on the cell plasma membrane or within the extracellular matrix, including collagen, gelatin, proteoglycans core protein, fibronectin, laminin and elastin. An imbalance between activated matrix metalloproteinases and their host-derived endogenous inhibitors leads to pathological breakdown of the extracellular matrix during periodontitis and numerous other diseases. Compensating for the deficit in the naturally occurring inhibitors or tissue inhibitors of matrix metalloproteinases to block or retard the proteolytic destruction of connective tissues is of therapeutic significance.

C) **PRO-INFLAMMATORY CYTOKINES**

Cytokines are defined as regulatory proteins controlling the survival, growth, differentiation and functions of cells. The term cytokine, meaning "cell protein," is reserved for molecules which transmit information or signals from one cell to another. It is part of a fundamental, cell-to-cell communication network. The term "paracrine" refers to signaling between different cell types usually in the same local environment. "Autocrine" refers to signaling between similar cell types or on "self." Interleukins (i.e, "proteins between leukocytes") refer to a special subgroup of cytokines which carry complex and often detailed messages or instructions between leukocytes, the white blood cells which comprise the immune system.

Cytokines are produced transiently at generally low concentrations, act and are degraded in a local environment. This is documented by the fact that cytokine-producing cells are often physically located immediately adjacent to the responding cells. Moreover, the responding cell destroys the cytokine that it responds to in the process of receptor-mediated endocytosis.

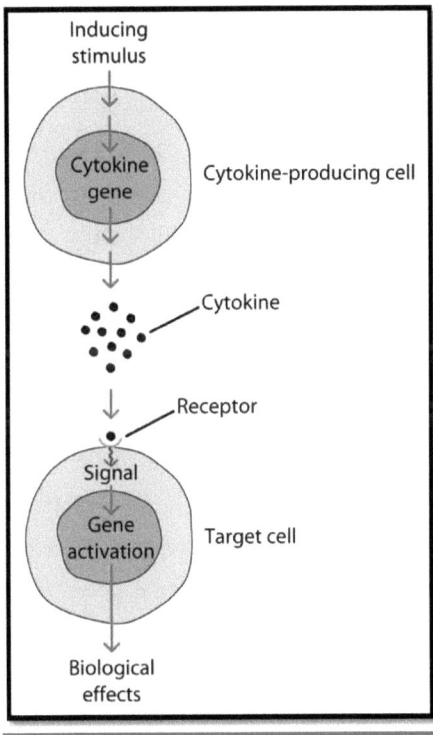

Fig.1. Mechanism of cytokine action on target cell

Interleukin-1, Interleukin-6 and tumor necrosis factor have all been found to be significantly elevated in diseased periodontal sites compared with healthy or inactive sites.[53,56] Interleukin-1 has also been positively correlated with increased probing depth and attachment loss.[56] Other clinical data indicate that elevated interleukin-6 levels are higher in refractory periodontitis.[57] Based upon the increased expression of IL-1, IL-6 and TNF in inflamed gingiva and high levels in the GCF of periodontitis patients, several studies have suggested that increased production of these cytokines may play an important role in periodontal tissue destruction.[10]

Interleukin -1

Interleukin -1 (IL-I) is a proinflammatory cytokine that has a large array of biological activities and directly regulates several genes expressed during inflammation.[58] There are 2 principal forms of interleukin-I that have agonist activity, IL-1α and IL-1β, with a third ligand, IL-1 receptor antagonist (lL-1ra) that functions as a competitive inhibitor. IL -lα and -β typically have similar activities. The biologic effects of IL-l have been implicated in the pathogenesis of several disease processes including asthma, congestive heart failure, arthritis, septic shock, and preterm labor (Okada S, 1995; Dudley D, 1997).[59,60] There are several lines of evidence that implicate IL-1 in the pathogenesis of periodontal disease as well. IL-1 is produced by several types of cells found in the periodontium and is elevated at sites with periodontal disease.[61]

Tumor Necrosis Factor

Tumor Necrosis Factor (TNF) refers to 2 associated proteins, TNF-α and lymphotoxin-alpha, also known as TNF-β. TNF-α is an inflammatory cytokine that is released by activated monocytes, macrophages and T lymphocytes, and promotes critical inflammatory responses during periodontal disease. High levels of TNF-α are extremely toxic to the host and it has been termed as 'suicide hormone'. The hypersecretion of TNF-α in diabetes, as observed both in GCF and by peripheral blood monocytic responses to LPS, has been proposed to be a contributing factor for increased severity of periodontal disease expression.[62] In vitro experiments have demonstrated that TNF-β may be cytotoxic for cultures of human gingival fibroblasts.[62]

Interleukin-6

Interleukin-6 (IL-6) is a major mediator of the host response to tissue injury and infection control.[63] Interleukin 6 is a product of lymphocytes, fibroblasts, and monocytes. Gingival fibroblast associated IL-6 has been observed by immunocytology in inflamed tissues.[64]

To prevent an uncontrolled inflammatory response with rapid tissue destruction, the activities of IL-1 and TNF-ά are naturally counteracted by the production of cytokines such as IL-4, IL-10 and IL-11.[65] More specifically, IL-11 has been shown to inhibit the production of IL-1ß, TNF- ά, IL-12 and nitric oxide (NO) in a variety of inflammatory conditions.[66]

D) PRODUCTION OF NITRIC OXIDE

Recently, Nitric Oxide (NO) has been shown to be a vital molecule in inflammatory processes.[15] Nitric oxide is synthesized from L-arginine by nitric oxide synthase (NOS), which is present in various tissues.[14]

There are three forms of nitric oxide synthases :
1) Type1 Nitric oxide synthase- brain enzyme (bNOS)
2) Type2 Nitric oxide synthase- inducible enzyme (iNOS), found in macrophages
3) Type3 Nitric oxide synthase- endothelial cell enzyme (eNOS)

eNOS and bNOS are named as constitutive NOS (cNOS) and produce modest levels of NO for a short period. Conversely, iNOS is expressed upon stimulation by proinflammatory mediators, such as IL-1β, TNF-α, interferon-γ.[67] eNOS causes vasodilatation. However macrophage derived iNOS is of interest; when released simultaneously with superoxide it forms reactive nitrogen species which is believed to be responsible for many of the cytotoxic effects.[67]

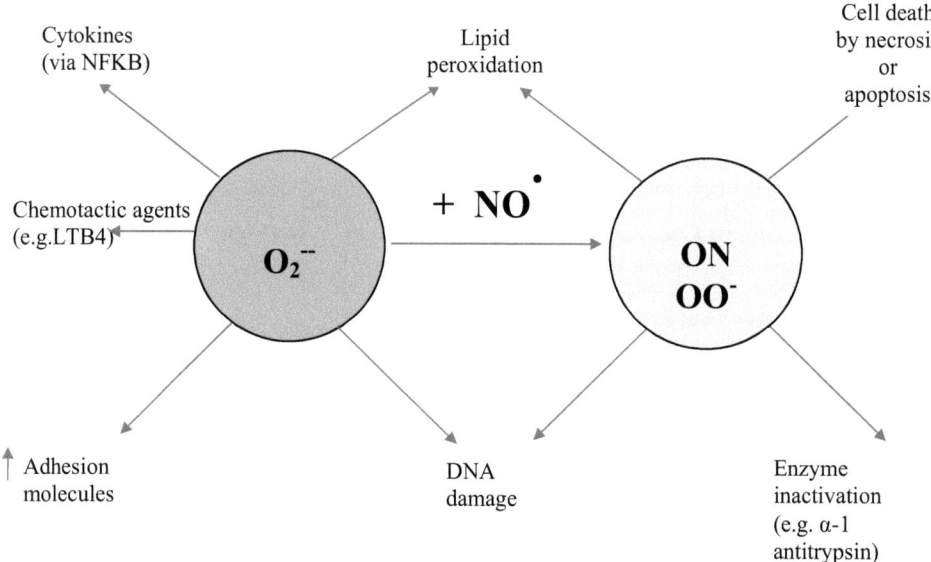

Fig.5. Interactions between superoxide & nitric oxide & their cellular effects.

It is known that NO is involved in acute and chronic inflammation.[14] Accumulating evidence from basic and clinical research suggests that NO may play a key role in mediating tissue and bone damage in inflammatory conditions associated with cytokine activation. It has been shown that NO activates matrix metalloproteins (MMPs)[68] ,and down- regulates synthesis of tissue inhibitors of matrix metal proteinases.[69] Local concentration of NOS is an essential determinant of cytotoxicity.

In recent years, a growing number of researchers have explored the role of NO in the pathophysiology of periodontal disease. Matejka et al[70] have shown increased NO synthesis in inflamed gingival tissues of patients with periodontal disease. Enhanced production of nitric oxide has been demonstrated in periodontal disease.[70]

E) REGULATION OF BONE REMODELING

It has long been accepted that bone formation and bone resorption are processes that are "coupled," although periodically there is evidence suggesting they can act independently.71 This coupling process entails that osteoclasts resorb an area of bone, and osteoblasts are signaled to come in and replace bone.

There are 2 molecules considered essential and sufficient to support osteoclastogenesis:
1) Macrophage colony-stimulating factor (M-CSF or CSF- I).
2) Receptor activator of nuclear factor kappa B ligand (RANKL).

RANKL is also known as osteoprotegerin-ligand, OPG-L, or TRANCE) is a cell surface protein present on osteoblastic cells and is responsible for osteoclast differentiation and bone.72 RANKL interacts with its receptor, RANK, on hematopoietic cells for differentiation and maturation of osteoclast precursor cells to activate osteoclasts. Osteoprotegerin acts as a decoy receptor, expressed by osteoblastic cells, which binds to RANKL and inhibits osteoclast development. Teng et al. (2000)73 showed that there is a strong evidence that RANKL/ OPG-L contributes to bone resorption in LJP.

There are relatively fewer inhibitors of bone resorption than stimulators of resorption. A soluble factor, osteoprotegerin (OPG) 73, binds to RANKL and inhibits the differentiation of osteoclasts. Interferon y16 is a cytokine produced by activated T lymphocytes that inhibits bone resorption by inhibiting the differentiation of committed precursors to mature cells.

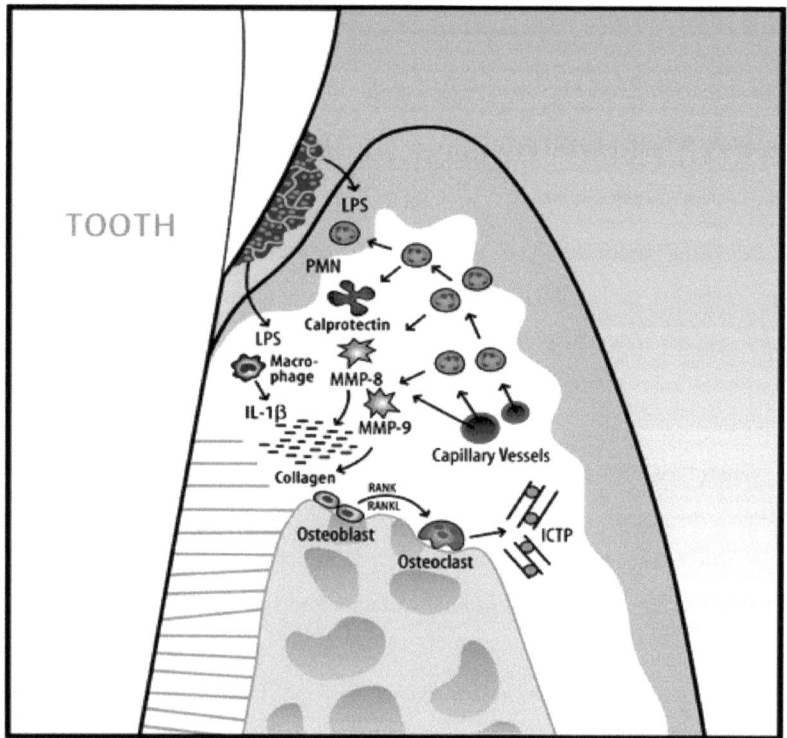

Fig.6. Schematic overview of the key biomarkers related to periodontal disease progression.

There is no doubt that plaque bacteria are necessary to initiate disease and drive the chronic inflammatory response in the periodontal tissues. At the same time there is strong evidence that destructive processes occurring as part of the host inflammatory response are responsible for the majority of the hard and soft tissue breakdown leading to the clinical signs of periodontitis. The characteristic clinical signs of chronic periodontitis occur mainly as a result of activation of host derived immune and inflammatory defense mechanism.

The transition process from gingival health to early inflammatory changes in response to bacterial challenge is characterized by the recruitment and activation of polymorphonuclear leukocytes (PMNs). In homeostasis, neutralization and phagocytosis of the invading microorganisms and secretion of appropriate cytokines may lead to a successful outcome of the inflammatory response. However, the outcome of host response may be destructive if elevated amounts of pro-inflammatory mediators, and enzymes are released. These include cytokines such as Interleukins and tumor necrosis factor, metabolites of the arachidonic acid pathway and matrix metalloproteinases (MMPs). Production of nitric oxide and regulation of bone remodeling also play key roles in pathogenesis of periodontal diseases.

The importance of host inflammatory response in the pathogenesis of periodontal diseases presents the opportunity to explore new treatment strategies. The adjunctive use of host modulation therapy with mechanical periodontal therapy has been reported involving non-surgical and surgical approaches.

HOST MODULATION THERAPY

The treatment strategies for periodontal disease have long been based on the understanding that plaque bacteria and their products primarily mediated the tissue destruction in affected patients. Therefore, the mechanical removal of dental plaque and calculus from tooth surfaces is considered the standard treatment for chronic periodontitis. Despite spectacular advances in medical sciences, treatment of periodontal diseases has changed very little, in principle, over the years. Scaling and root planning (SRP) remains the "gold standard" treatment for periodontitis against which other treatments are compared. Moreover, the clinical improvements that can be expected to occur following SRP are remarkably consistent across studies. Thus, periodontal treatment through the ages has focused on the reduction of bacterial infection by mechanical removal of infectious agents (i.e. SRP).

To date, non-surgical periodontal treatment has primarily focused on reducing the bacterial burden by mechanical disruption of the subgingival biofilm by SRP. Locally delivered topical antimicrobial agents are also used together with SRP to further reduce the bacterial burden. There is no doubt that plaque bacteria are necessary to initiate disease and drive the chronic inflammatory response in the periodontal tissues. Recent research into the pathogenesis of periodontal diseases has led to an important paradigm shift in the way we view periodontal disease progression. It is now recognized that the major component of the soft and hard tissue destruction seen in periodontitis occurs as a result of activation of the host's immune-inflammatory defense mechanisms in response to the presence of bacterial plaque. The development of host modulatory therapies, together with our better understanding of risk factors and disease processes allows us now to improve upon the age old treatment strategy of root surface debridement.

The importance of the host inflammatory response in periodontal pathogenesis presents the opportunity for exploiting new treatment strategies for periodontitis by means of host response modulation. With this current understanding of the host response and periodontal disease pathogenesis, it is intuitive that pharmaceutical inhibition of host response pathways may be an adjunctive or alternative strategy for treating periodontal diseases. Host modulatory therapy (HMT) can be combined with traditional periodontal therapies that reduce the bacterial burden (e.g. SRP) to constitute a comprehensive treatment strategy for periodontitis.

The host inflammatory response in periodontal pathogenesis include production of arachidonic acid metabolites, matrix metalloproteinases, cytokines, nitric oxide and mediators of periodontal osseous remodeling. Therefore, clinical utility of therapeutic modulation of host response in the management of periodontal disease is reviewed under following headings: modulation of arachidonic acid metabolites, modulation of host matrix metalloproteinases, modulation of host cytokines, modulation of nitric oxide activity and modulation of bone remodeling

A) **MODULATION OF ARACHIDONIC ACID METABOLITES**

Arachidonic acid is liberated from membrane phospholipids of the cells after tissue damage or stimulus by the action of enzyme phospholipase and is metabolized via either the cyclooxygenase (COX) or the lipooxygenase (LO) pathways. The cyclooxygenase pathway produces prostaglandins, prostacyclin and thromboxane called prostanoids, while lipooxygenase pathway forms the leukotrienes (LTs) and other monohydroxy-eicosatetraenoic acids. The cyclooxygenase enzymes are recognized to have two isoforms.

Cyclooxygenase-1 (COX-1) which is a constitutive enzyme expressed in mast cells and tissues, and appears to represent an essential component of tissue homeostasis. In contrast, COX-2 which is inducible and is present in cells involved in the inflammatory process.[18] It is upregulated by IL-1β, TNF-α, bacteria and lipopolysaccharide (LPS).[134,19] Cells stimulated with cytokines such as IL-1β or LPS are able to rapidly synthesize COX-2 from pr1e-existing mRNA and translate new COX-2 transcripts, leading to a prolonged COX-2 release without inducing COX-1 biosynthesis.

Some prostanoids have pro-inflammatory properties and have been associated with destructive processes in inflammatory disease. In bone organ culture, PGE_2 stimulates osteoclastic bone resorption.[135] PGE_2 is a potent inducer of MMP secretion by monocytes and fibroblasts to trigger connective tissue destruction.[22] PGE_2 interacts synergistically with IL-1 and TNF-α to enhance the effects of these molecules. In periodontal disease, prostaglandin E_2 has been extensively co-related with inflammation and bone resorption.[23]

I) *Non Steroidal Anti Inflammatory Drugs (NSAIDS)*

Role of cyclooxygenase in progression of periodontal disease has been studied to an enormous extent & it has been evident that cyclooxygenase play a role in progression of periodontal disease. Since then, numerous studies have been conducted in animals and humans using non-steriodal anti-inflammatory drugs (NSAIDs) to block the prostanoid production by inhibiting cyclooxygenases. The majority of NSAIDs are weak organic acids that selectively (COX-2) and non-selectively (COX-1) inhibit the synthesis of arachidonic acid metabolites, thereby blocking the production of prostaglandins, thromboxane and prostacyclin.

Heasman et.al (1993)[78] examined the **effects of a potent cyclooxygenase inhibitor, flurbiprofen, on both clinical parameters and on release of PGE_2, TxB_2 and LTB_4 during the development of inflammation using the**

experimental gingivitis model in 21 humans. They also studied the effects of the drug on established gingivitis. 7 subjects were prescribed flurbiprofen, 50 mg bid for 21 days while placebo was prescribed for 14 subjects. Gingival redness and bleeding on probing were assessed at baseline, 7, 14 and 21 days. Gingival Crevicular fluid (GCF) samples were also collected to determine concentrations of PGE_2, TxB_2 and LTB_4 at baseline and at 21 days. The flurbiprofen significantly inhibited the development of redness and bleeding effects, which were associated with a significant inhibition of TxB_2. However it did not effect the concentration of GCF- PGE_2 or GCF-LTB_4 during this 21-day gingivitis, model. To assess the effects of flurbiprofen on established experimental gingivitis, this study was extended to 28 days on the same model. On day 21, the placebo group was subdivided into 2 groups of 7 subjects each. One group was prescribed flurbiprofen (50 mg b.d.) for 7 days and controls (C2) continued to take placebo. All subjects continued to abstain from tooth cleaning. Pretreatment (day 21) and post-treatment (day 28) comparisons showed that flurbiprofen again significantly inhibited bleeding, but did not affect redness. Control subjects demonstrated a significant elevation in gingival bleeding on day 28, and this was associated with significant rises in GCF-PGE_2, GCF-TxB_2 and GCF-LTB_4. The authors reported that **flurbiprofen controls gingival inflammation at both preventive and therapeutic levels** in the experimental gingivitis model and suggested that this effect could be associated with an inhibition in the production of cyclooxygenase metabolites that indirectly affects GCF- LTB_4 levels.

Jeffcoat et al (1995)[80] assessed the **efficacy of a topical NSAID rinse, containing ketorolac tromethamine** as the active agent. 55 adult periodontitis patients were studied in this 6-month randomized, double blind, parallel, placebo and positive-controlled study. Patients were divided into three groups: 1) bid ketorolac rinse (0.1%) with placebo capsule; 2) 50 mg bid flurbiprofen capsule (positive control) with placebo rinse; or 3) bid placebo rinse and capsule. Prophylaxes were provided every 3 months. Monthly examinations assessed safety, gingival condition, and gingival crevicular fluid PGE_2. Standardized radiographs were taken at baseline, at 3 and at 6 months by digital subtraction radiography. A significant loss in bone height was observed during the study period in the placebo group (-0.63 ± 0.11), but not in the flurbiprofen (-0.10 ± 0.12) or ketorolac rinse (+0.20 ± 0.11 mm) groups. It was found that ketorolac and flurbiprofen groups had less bone loss and reduced gingival crevicular fluid PGE2 levels compared to placebo. It was concluded that ketorolac rinse preserved more alveolar bone than systemic flurbiprofen and that **ketorolac rinse may be beneficial in the treatment of adult periodontitis.**

Preshaw et.al (1998)[81] investigated the effects of topical ketorolac tromethamine mouthrinse (0.1%) on gingival crevicular fluid (GCF) prostaglandin E_2 (PGE_2) concentrations. This study was conducted for 6 weeks interval & was a randomized double blind, placebo controlled, parallel group study. The study enrolled a total of 42 patients with moderately advanced adult periodontitis. GCF samples were collected & measured using immunoassay kit. This study concluded that ketorolac mouth rinse controlled the elevation of GCF PGE2 compared to placebo, but did not actually reduced GCF PGE2 concentrations

Bezerra M. (2000)[84] compared the **effect of a selective COX-2 inhibitors – meloxicam and indomethacin- on alveolar bone loss (ABL)** in an experimental periodontitis model in rats. 48 Wistar rats were subjected to placement of a nylon thread ligature around the maxillary molars and sacrificed after 7 days. Alveolar bone loss (ABL) was measured in one quadrant as the distance between the cemento-enamel junction and the alveolar bone. The other quadrant was processed for histopathologic analysis. Daily weight and white blood cell count were recorded. Groups were treated subcutaneously for 7 days with either IND (0.5, 1, or 2 mg/kg) or MLX (0.75, 1.5, or 3 mg/kg). Controls received no treatment. Macroscopic analysis of the gastric mucosa was done. The control group did not receive any manipulation, and a non-treated group consisted of rats subjected to periodontitis that received no pharmacological treatment. The results showed that in the non-treated (NT) group, there was significant ABL, severe mononuclear influx, and an increase in osteoclast numbers. Significant neutrophilia and lymphomonocytosis occurred at 6 hours and at 7 days, respectively, as compared to controls. Significant weight loss persisted until the seventh day in the NT group. Both IND and MLX reduced ABL and histopathologic changes. Neutrophilia and lymphomonocytosis were also significantly reversed. Both IND and MLX induced earlier weight recovery. The stomachs of the IND (1 and 2 mg/kg) groups presented hemorrhage and ulcers, whereas in the MLX-treated groups, there were mild petechiae that was seen only in the 3 mg/kg group. The authors suggested that both **indomethacin and meloxicam prevented ABL and reduced inflammatory changes through COX inhibition.** They also observed that meloxicam displays similar efficacy and less gastric damage than indomethacin.

Holzhausen et.al (2002)[86] conducted a study which evaluated **the effect of a selective cyclooxygenase-2 inhibitor (celecoxib) on alveolar bone resorption** in experimentally induced periodontal disease in 180 wistar rats by placing cotton ligatures at the gingival margin level. The rats were randomly assigned to one of the following groups that received: a daily oral dose of 10 mg/kg body weight of celecoxib (Ce1); 20 mg/kg body weight of celecoxib (Ce2); or 10 ml/kg of saline solution (C). Serum levels of celecoxib and white blood cell count were determined. Standardized digital radiographs were obtained after sacrificing at 3, 5, 10, 18, and 30 days to measure the amount of bone loss around the mesial root surface of the first molar tooth in each rat. The results showed that **groups treated with celecoxib had significantly less bone loss compared to control group** and that there has been a significant interaction between treatment with celecoxib and time. Comparisons showed that in both the groups treated with celecoxib, the bone loss became significant only after 10 days of ligature placement, while in the control group it was already significant after 5 days. However, there was no significant difference in bone loss among experimental groups at the end of the experimental period. It was concluded that the systemic therapy with the celecoxib could modify the progression of experimentally induced periodontitis in rats.

Gurgel et.al (2004)[89] investigated the **impact of a selective cyclooxygenase-2 inhibitor (meloxicam) on bone loss** in ligature-induced periodontitis and its post-treatment effect after its administration withdrawal in seventy-five adult male Wistar rats. After anesthesia, a mandibular first molar was randomly assigned to receive the cotton ligature, while the contra lateral tooth was left unligated. The animals were randomly assigned to one of the following five treatment groups (15 animals each), by daily subcutaneous injections of: 1) saline solution for 15 days; 2) saline solution for 45 days; 3) 3 mg/kg of meloxicam for 15 days; 4) 3 mg/kg of meloxicam for 45 days; or 5) 3 mg/kg of meloxicam for 15 days followed by saline solution for 30 days. The animals were sacrificed and the specimens were routinely processed. The volume of bone loss was histometrically measured. Intergroup comparisons demonstrated that the drug significantly reduced periodontitis-related bone loss (group 3: 5.83 +/- 2.04); however, this effect was less evident when the drug was administered in a short period (group 4: 3.59 +/- 1.57). Moreover, after drug withdrawal, no residual effect was observed (6.86 +/- 3.59, 6.09 +/- 2.66, groups 2 and 5, respectively). The authors concluded that selective cyclooxygenase-2 inhibitors may reduce bone loss associated with experimental periodontitis and that there is no remaining effect after its withdrawal.

Paquette et.al (2000)[85] evaluated the pharmacodynamic **effects of the NSAID, ketoprofen on gingival crevicular fluid (GCF) prostanoids.** 42

subjects, ages 35-57 years, with moderate to advanced adult periodontitis were recruited and monitored for 22 days. On day 1, subjects were randomized for 1 of 5 treatments: i) 0.5% ketoprofen gel; ii) 1.0% ketoprofen gel; iii) 1.0% ketoprofen alternate gel; iv) 2.0% ketoprofen gel; v) 25 mg ketoprofen capsule (positive control). Subjects had applied 1 ml of gel topically to their gingiva or administered one capsule, bid for 14.5 days. GCF samples were collected from posterior, interproximal sites on days 1 (pre-dosing; 1, 2, 3, 6 h), 8 (pre-dosing; 2 h), 15 (pre-dosing; 2 h) and 22 (post-treatment). GCF levels of prostaglandin E_2 (PGE_2) and leukotriene B_4 (LTB_4) were determined using RIA, and expressed in ng/ml and % reduction from baseline (%Effect). When data was combined from all groups, significant % of reductions in GCF PGE_2 were noted at 1 and 2 h post-dosing (29% and 24% respectively). In comparing topical versus systemic formulations, all topical formulations were as equipotent as systemic dosing in altering local prostaglandin levels despite lower ketoprofen exposures with gel treatments. These authors concluded that both **topical and systemic ketoprofen therapies pharmacodynamically reduce GCF PGE_2 levels in adult periodontitis subjects resulting in inhibition of disease progression.**

S. Atilla et.al (2002)[136] conducted a study which was aimed at evaluating the **effects of adjunctive meloxicam on matrix metalloproteinase-8 (MMP-8) levels of gingival crevicular fluid (GCF) following initial phase of periodontal therapy .**A total 12 patients having chronic periodontitis were enrolled into this study. Patients received 7.5 mg meloxicam, and 10 patients received placebo tablets together with scaling and root planing in a 1 x 1 regimen for 10 days. Scaling and root planing were performed on day 3 of drug intake. The MMP-8 levels in GCF samples obtained before and on day 10 of drug intake were determined by using the immunofluorescence assay. Plaque index (PI), papilla bleeding index (PBI), and GCF MMP-8 levels were recorded. Both meloxicam and placebo groups showed statistically significant reductions in PBI, PI, and GCF MMP-8 levels on day 10 compared to baseline. The GCF MMP-8 level on day 10 in the meloxicam group was similar to the clinically healthy control group, while it was significantly higher in the placebo group. Positive correlations were found between MMP-8 total amounts and PBI scores at baseline and day 10 of drug intake in the patient groups. **Meloxicam showed a tendency to reduce GCF MMP-8 levels** within the first 10 days, when used as an adjunct in the initial phase of periodontal treatment. Based on these findings the authors suggested that adjunctive use of selective COX-2 inhibitor is beneficial in treatment of chronic periodontitis patients.

Vardar et.al (2003)[87] compared the effects of selective cyclooxygenase (COX)-2 inhibitor (nimesulide) and non-selective COX-1/COX-2 inhibitor (naproxen) as an adjunct to non-surgical (SRP) periodontal therapy in chronic periodontitis patients on the gingival tissue levels of prostaglandin PGE_2 and $PGF_{2\alpha}$. A total of thirty patients with chronic periodontitis (17 males and 13 females; aged 35 to 59 years) were divided into 3 groups of 10 patients each. One group received 100 mg of nimesulide; second group received 275 mg of naproxen sodium; and the third group received placebo tablets for 10 days as an adjunct to SRP. The periodontal status was determined by measuring Probing depth (PD), Clinical attachment level (CAL), Plaque index (PI) and papillary bleeding index (PBI) at baseline, and at 3 months. The levels of PGE_2 were detected using an enzyme immunoassay (EIA), while the levels of PGF_2 were analyzed by radioimmunoassay (RIA). Gingival tissue samples were obtained before drug intake and on day 10. All 3 groups showed statistically significant reductions in PBI, PI, PD and CAL at 3 months. Both the nimesulide and naproxen groups showed a significant decrease in PGF_2 level, while the placebo group showed a significant increase. The authors concluded that nimesulide may have additional inhibitory effects on gingival tissue $PGF_{2\alpha}$ levels in the first week following non-surgical periodontal treatment. However, it has an insignificant effect on reducing PGE_2 levels in gingival tissue.

Kurtis et.al (2007)[91] investigated the effect of systemic flurbiprofen administration as an adjunct to SRP on clinical parameters, PGE_2 and thiobarbituric acid reactive substance (TBARS) levels in gingival crevicular fluid (GCF) samples from smoker and non-smoker patients with chronic periodontitis. A total of 42 subjects were divided into following 4 groups: Group 1: ten non-smokers with chronic periodontitis (CP). Periodontal treatment: SRP plus systemic NSAID (flurbiprofen tablet, 100 mg; twice daily for 10 days). Group 2: eleven non-smokers with CP. Periodontal treatment: SRP plus placebo tablets (Twice daily for 10 days). Group 3. Ten smokers with CP. Periodontal treatment: SRP plus systemic NSAID (Flurbiprofen tablet, 100 mg;twice daily for 10 days). Group 4. Eleven smokers with CP. Periodontal treatment: SRP plus placebo tablets (Twice daily for 10 days). GCF samples were collected at baseline and on day 10 of drug intake from each sampling area by a single examiner, who was unaware of the treatment modality. The levels of PGE2 and TBARS in GCF samples were carried out by an enzyme-linked immunosorbent assay and fluorometric method, respectively. PI and GI scores were decreased after therapy in all groups following the phase I periodontal treatment on day 10, but no statistical differences were observed in PD and CAL scores after the therapy. In groups 1 and 2, the reduction of GCF PGE_2 and TBARS levels were not significant after the therapy compared to baseline levels. In group 3, GCF PGE_2 and TBARS levels exhibited a statistically significant decrease after the therapy. Group 4 showed significant reductions in GCF PGE_2 levels after the therapy. No statistically significant reductions were observed in group 4 with regard to GCF TBARS levels. When groups 1 and 3 were compared for GCF TBARS levels after the therapy, a more statistically significant reduction was observed in group 3. The authors concluded that better results for GCF PGE_2 and TBARS levels in smokers compared to non-smokers can be attributed to the differences in synergistic effects of combined flurbiprofen and SRP between smokers and non-smokers.

Sekino et.al (2005)[90] conducted a study on eleven subjects to **evaluate the effect of systemic administration of ibuprofen on gingivitis and de novo plaque formation.** Subjects were given oral hygiene instruction, scaling and professional mechanical tooth cleaning. At the end of a preparatory period (Day 0), the participants were told to abstain from all mechanical plaque control measures during a 2-week experimental period but to rinse with an assigned mouth rinse, for positive control: 0.1% chlorhexidine digluconate and for negative control: saline or administer ibuprofen tablets of 200 mg twice daily. Mouth rinsing was performed twice a day, for 60 seconds with 10 ml. Re-examination was performed after 14 days of experiment. After a 2-week "wash-out" period, the participants received a new mechanical tooth cleaning and a second 14-day experimental period was initiated. The experimental and "wash-out" periods were repeated until all volunteers had been involved in all three regimens. Supragingival plaque was collected and prepared for dark-field microscopy. One hundred bacterial cells were counted and classified into six different groups: coccoid cells, straight rods, filaments, fusiforms, spirochetes and motile rods. Gingival crevicular fluid (GCF) was collected from the same sites that were sampled for plaque. The volume of GCF collected in each strip was measured and analyzed regarding content of lactoferrin and albumin. It was observed that during the period when the subjects rinsed with saline they accumulated large amounts of plaque and developed marked signs of gingivitis. When they rinsed with chlorhexidine digluconate, small amounts of plaque formed and few sites received GI score ≥ 2. After the 2 weeks of ibuprofen administration, the subjects presented with significantly fewer sites that scored GI ≥ 2 but had formed similar amounts of plaque as during the negative control period. **The authors concluded that ibuprofen administered via the systemic route has an effect on gingivitis but not on de novo plaque formation.**

Heasman et.al (1994)[79] conducted a study which was aimed at investigating the effect of a systemic flurbiprofen preparation (100 mg daily) on the resolution of experimental gingivitis in 47 human volunteers. The subjects were then given a course of scaling, polishing and oral hygiene instruction to achieve a healthy gingival status at baseline. The subjects then abstained from cleaning their mouth for 21 days. On day 21 each subject was allocated randomly to receive one of the two treatments. Treatment A (23 subjects): flurbiprofen tablet (50 mg, twice daily) + toothbrushing. Treatment B (24 subjects): placebo tablet (twice daily) + toothbrushing. Each treatment was continued for 7 days. Plaque indices, gingival indices and GCF flow were assessed at baseline, on day 21 and 27. There was no significant difference between the group for plaque indices or GCF flow. The flurbiprofen group, however, demonstrated greater resolution of gingival inflammation by day 27 when compared to the placebo control. The GCF flow was also reduced significantly in each group between days 21 and 27. Inter-group analysis indicated that although the magnitude of the reduction was greater in the flurbiprofen group, but the difference was not statistically significant. **The authors concluded that the flurbiprofen has a beneficial effect by increasing the rate of resolution of inflammation.**

Heasman et.al (1989)[75] investigated the effects of a topical NSAID solution (flurbiprofen - a phenylalkenoic acid and potent cyclooxygenase inhibitor) on the development of experimentally-induced gingivitis in human. 24 healthy volunteers abstained from tooth-cleaning for 17 days. Parameters of gingival health were recorded on days 1 and 17. On days 4, 6, 8, 11, 13 and 15, each volunteer randomly received, on a double-blind basis 100 ml of 10 mM flurbiprofen solution in buffered preservative to one upper quadrant of the mouth using a pulsed Jet irrigating system. The contralateral quadrant received preservative only. When gingival health was re-established, 4 volunteer, had further 3 irrigation, of flurbiprofen at intervals of 2 days. Plasma levels of flurbiprofen were determined after the 1st and 3rd irrigation. Assays showed that the drug was present in the plasma of all 4 subjects (range 0.2-0. 7 µg/ml). Gingival health was re-established in 6 further volunteers from the original study. They then abstained from tooth brushing for 17 days, during which one maxillary quadrant was irrigated with the buffered preservative solution. The irrigation, were made on the same basis as in the original study. Gingivitis again developed in these quadrants, although when the results were compared to the equivalent data from the first investigation, significantly greater median values for probing pocket depth, and gingival indices were found in the latter study. The authors concluded that systemic absorption of flurbiprofen reduces the severity of developing inflammatory lesion.

Fieldman et.al (1983)[74] investigated the effect of non-steroidal anti-inflammatory drugs on the alveolar bone levels in 75 patients with a long term history of aspirin and/or indomethacin therapy with the help of dental radiographs and medical records. Patients were selected on the basis of aspirin and/or indomethacin therapy for at least 5 previous consecutive years (ASA group). The ASA study group was matched according to age and similarity of remaining dentition with a comparison group of 75 male volunteers (DLS group). Both groups received a comprehensive dental evaluation including a full mouth IOPA radiographs. The amount of bone remaining around each tooth, as visualized on dental radiographs, was measured with a 10 point Schei ruler. In the ASA group, the mean number of sites with bone loss was 33.17 (76.7%), while the mean number of bone loss sites was 37.27 (82.2%) for the DLS group. The mean percentage of bone loss was also lower for the ASA group (14.2%), as compared to the DLS control (15.8%); however, the difference was not statistically significant. Therefore, it was concluded that the inhibition of bone loss found in their study could be due to the chronic ingestion of ASA or ASA and indomethacin.

Williams et.al (1989)[76] studied the effect of the NSAID, flurbiprofen in fifty-six individuals with radiographic evidence of alveolar bone loss. Following a 6 month baseline pretreatment period to measure the radiographic progression of bone loss, half of the patients were administered flurbiprofen, 50 mg. bid., while half were administered a placebo. All patients received a subgingival scaling and pumice by a hygienist every 6 months. The rate of alveolar bone loss in 2 year treatment period was compared to the baseline 6 month pretreatment period within and between patient groups. In individuals given placebo tablets, the rate of bone loss was significantly less than baseline at 6 and 12 months of treatment, but not thereafter. Individuals given flurbiprofen twice daily had a significant decrease in rate of bone loss compared to baseline at 6, 12 and 18 months of treatment. At 12 and 18 months the rate of bone loss in the flurbiprofen treated individuals was significantly less than in the placebo patients. However at 24 months of the treatment period, there was no difference in the rate of bone loss between the placebo and flurbiprofen treated patients. The authors concluded that the NSAID flurbiprofen, as an inhibitor, of cyclooxygenase, can inhibit human alveolar bone loss as measured radiographically.

Reddy et.al (1993)[77] studied the effect of the non-steroidal anti-inflammatory drug, **meclofenamate sodium (Meclomen), as an adjunct to scaling and root planing on the progression of alveolar bone loss associated with rapidly progressive periodontitis (RPP).** 22 subjects (7 male, 15 female) of mean age of 36.5 years with disease-active RPP by pretreatment bone scan with standardized radiographs at baseline and at 6 months. Following full-mouth scaling and root planing, subjects were randomly assigned to either a placebo, "Low-dose" (50mg) or "High-dose" 100 mg meclofenamate sodium bid group. Bone change over the 6-month period as assessed by subtraction radiography was the primary efficacy determinant. The results revealed a significant dose response, with the placebo group having a mean bone loss of 0.42 mm, low and high dose groups having mean bone gains of 0.07 and 0.20 mm, respectively. Based on these findings the authors concluded that **meclofenamate sodium may have a potential role in treatment regimens for patients with rapidly progressive periodontitis.**

Bichara et.al (1999)[82] studied the effect of a one week course of postsurgical naproxen (500mg, twice daily for one week) on the osseous healing in intrabony defects treated with polylactide bioabsorbable membranes. Twenty-four vertical osseous defects in 24 patients (12 males, 12 females [age 37 to 72 years; mean 44 years]) were treated with either a bioabsorbable membrane plus twice daily postsurgical naproxen 500 mg for one week (test group) or with a polylactide bioabsorbable membrane alone (control group). Treatment was performed on 12 patients either with 2- or 3-wall or combination defects without any adjunctive root conditioning or bone graft. Open defect measurements from baseline to 9 months showed a statistically significant mean defect fill of 1.96 ± 1.27 mm and 2.04 ± 1.71 for the test (GPN) and control (GA) groups, respectively. This corresponded to a mean defect fill of 42% and a mean defect resolution of approximately 75% for both groups. The differences between GPN and GA groups were not statistically significant. Defect fill of ≥ 50% was seen in 6 defects (50%) in the test group and in 5 defects (42%) in the control group. An administration of postsurgical naproxen did not produce superior defect fill compared to that obtained with polylactide bioabsorbable membranes alone.

Thais M. Oliveira et al (2008)[93] evaluated the **effect of a preferential cyclooxygenase (COX)-2 inhibitor meloxicam on VEGF expression and alveolar bone loss in experimentally induced periodontitis.** A total of 120 Wistar rats were randomly separated into groups 1 (control) and 2 (meloxicam, 3 mg/kg/day, intraperitoneally, for 3, 7, 14, or 30 days). Silk ligatures were placed at the gingival margin level of the lower right first molar of all rats. VEGF expression was assessed by reverse transcription-polymerase chain reaction (RT-PCR), Western blot (WB), and immunohistochemical (IHC) analyses. A reduction in alveolar bone resorption was observed in the meloxicam-treated group compared to the control group at all periods studied. Meloxicam significantly reduced the increased mRNA VEGF expression in diseased tissues after 14 days of treatment. VEGF protein expression in WB experiments was significantly higher in diseased sites compared to healthy sites. After 14 days of treatment with meloxicam, an important decrease in VEGF protein expression was detected in diseased tissues. Qualitative IHC analysis revealed that VEGF protein expression was higher in diseased tissues and decreased in tissues from rats treated with meloxicam. The present data suggest an important role for VEGF in the progression of periodontal disease. **Systemic therapy with meloxicam can modify the progression of experimentally induced periodontitis in rats by reducing VEGF expression and alveolar bone loss.**

C. Alec Yen et al (2008)[92] tested the **efficacy of celecoxib (COX-2 inhibitor) in conjunction with scaling and root planing (SRP) in subjects with chronic periodontitis (CP).** A total of 131 subjects were randomized to receive SRP and either celecoxib (200 mg) or placebo every day for 6 months. Clinical outcomes were assessed every 3 months for 12 months as mean changes from baseline. Primary efficacy parameters included clinical attachment level (CAL) and probing depth (PD). Secondary outcomes included percentages of tooth sites with CAL loss or gain ≥2 mm, changes in bleeding on probing (BOP), plaque index, and mobility. Prior to analysis, tooth sites were grouped based on baseline PD as shallow (1 to 3 mm), moderate (4 to 6 mm), or deep (≥7 mm). Mean PD reduction and CAL gain were greater in the celecoxib group, primarily in moderate and deep sites, throughout the study (PD: 3.84 mm versus 2.06 mm; CAL: 3.74 mm versus 1.43 mm, for deep sites at 12 months). The celecoxib group also exhibited a greater percentage of sites with ≥2 mm CAL gain and fewer sites with ≥2 mm CAL loss. This study concluded that **celecoxib can be an effective adjunctive treatment to SRP to reduce progressive attachment loss in subjects with CP.** Moreover, its beneficiary effect persisted even at 6 months post administration.

Various types of NSAIDs have been used with anti-inflammatory activity ranging from mild (e.g., aspirin) to potent (e.g., flurbiprofen, ketorolac), as an adjuvant to scaling, root planing and surgical procedures including guided tissue regeneration therapy either by systemic administration or by topical application. But the most frequently evaluated drug is flurbiprofen. **These investigations tend to consistently show a statistically significant benefit favoring use of adjunctive NSAIDs to periodontal therapy.** However, suppression of prostaglandin production, by NSAIDs may cause gastric ulceration by impairing the protective function of the mucosal barrier (Hawkey 1993)[137], renal failure (Lindsley & Warady 1990)[138] and cardiovascular risks (Wardle 2004).[139] While our understanding of the role of COX-2 in the pathogenesis of periodontitis suggests that inhibition of COX-2 might be a desirable target for therapeutic intervention, however serious adverse effects of current formulations preclude their use as an adjunct to periodontal therapy.

II) Lipoxins (LX) and Aspirin Triggered Lipoxins (ATL)

Recent evidence suggests that lipoxins (LX) are a class of both structurally and functionally unique eicosanoids involved in counter-regulation of inflammatory responses.[6] These lipid mediators also appear to facilitate the resolution of the acute inflammatory response.[139] LX and aspirin-triggered lipoxin (ATL) are bioactive lipid mediators involved in the Arachidonic acid cascade and are formed by the interaction of 5- and 15-LOs.[140] Like most lipid mediators, lipoxins are rapidly synthesized, act within a local environment and are rapidly enzymatically degraded. Metabolically stable analogues of both LXA4 and its epimer 15-epi LXA4 are involved in the resolution of inflammatory processes.[141]

Pouliot et.al (2000)[142] investigated the potential protective contribution of lipoxins in the murine air pouch model. Porphyromonas gingivalis was introduced within murine dorsal air pouches. In the air pouch cavity, P. gingivalis elicited leukocyte infiltration, concomitant with elevated PGE_2 levels in the cellular exudates, and up-regulated COX-2 expression in infiltrated leukocytes. In addition, human neutrophils exposed to P. gingivalis also upregulated COX-2 expression. The administration of metabolically stable analogues of LX and of aspirin-triggered LX potently blocked neutrophil traffic into the dorsal pouch cavity and lowered PGE_2 levels within exudates. The authors concluded that there was protective role of LX during inflammation in murine air pouch model limiting further PMN recruitment and PMN-mediated tissue injury.

Serhan et.al (2003)[88] examined transgenic (TG) rabbits over-expressing 15-LO type 1 and their response to inflammatory challenge. Skin challenges with either LTB_4 or IL-8 showed that 15-LO TG rabbits gave markedly reduced neutrophil (PMN) recruitment and plasma leakage at dermal sites with LTB_4. Leukocytes from 15-LO TG rabbits gave enhanced LX production, underscoring differences in lipid mediator profiles compared with non-TG rabbits. Microbe-associated inflammation and leukocyte-mediated bone destruction were assessed by initiating acute periodontitis. 15-LO TG rabbits exhibited markedly reduced bone loss and local inflammation. Enhanced LX production was associated with an increased anti-inflammatory status. Topical application with the 15-epi-16-phenoxy-para-fluoro-LXA_4 stable analog (ATLa) dramatically reduced leukocyte infiltration, ensuing bone loss as well as inflammation. The authors concluded **LXs can be targets for novel approaches to diseases, e.g., periodontitis and arthritis, where inflammation and bone destruction are features.**

Pouliot et.al (1999)[83] investigated the impact of metabolically stable LX and ATL analogues on TNF-α induced neutrophil response. At nanomolar levels, the LXA4 and ATL analog 15 R/S-methyl-LXA4 each blocked TNF α -stimulated IL-1 β release by isolated human PMN in vitro. The TNF α -induced IL-1 β gene expression was also regulated by 15 R/S-methyl-LXA4. In addition, 15 R/S-methyl-LXA4 added to murine air pouches dramatically inhibited TNF α -stimulated leukocyte trafficking in vivo, as well as altered the appearance of both macrophage inflammatory peptide-2 and IL-1 β and concomitantly stimulated IL-4 in pouch exudates. The **authors concluded that both LXA4 and ATL are regulators of TNF α -directed neutrophil actions and stimulate IL-4 to play an important role in preventing periodontal disease**.

Collectively, data from experimental animal studies have shown that **lipoxins are capable of preventing gingival inflammation and bone loss in animal experimental periodontitis.** However, further studies are necessary to determine the efficacy of these drugs and their potential role as a host modulation therapeutic agent.

B) MODULATION OF HOST MATRIX METALLOPROTEINASES

It is well established that bacterial plaque is essential for initiation of chronic periodontitis, but the characteristic clinical signs of chronic periodontitis occur mainly as a result of activation of host derived immune and inflammatory defense mechanism. The development of an immune-inflammatory response in the susceptible individual results in local production of a variety of pro-inflammatory mediators. Key among these are the matrix metalloproteinases which have the capacity to degrade all components of the extracellular matrix of the periodontium. MMPs are produced by each of the major cell types found in human periodontal tissues including fibroblasts, keratinocytes, macrophages, PMNs (neutrophils) and endothelial cells. In healthy tissues, MMPs are produced primarily by fibroblasts (MMP-1 or collagenase-1) and are concerned with the maintenance of the periodontal connective tissues.

Regulation of MMP activity involves specific, endogenous tissue inhibitors of MMPs (TIMPs) and α-macroglobulins, which form complexes with active MMPs, and in some cases with latent MMP precursors.[143,11] TIMPs are produced by various cell types including fibroblasts, keratinocytes, macrophages and endothelial cells and are widely distributed in body fluids and tissues.[45] Transcription of MMP genes is upregulated by pro-inflammatory mediators known to be important in periodontal disease progression, including interleukin- 1α and β (IL-1 α and β) and tumor necrosis factor- α (TNF- α).[47]

Collagen turnover in healthy tissues is a controlled intracellular event that is mediated extracellularly by fibroblast derived collagenase (MMP-1) and intracellularly by a variety of lysosomal acid-dependent enzymes. **In inflamed periodontal tissues, the balance between MMPs and TIMPs is disrupted as a result of pathological alterations in the types and quantities of MMPs present.** This leads to excessive breakdown of extracellular collagen and inappropriate destruction of periodontal tissues. There is increased secretion of **MMP-8** (neutrophil-derived collagenase, collagenase-2) and **MMP-9** (neutrophil derived gelatinase, gelatinase-B) by infiltrating PMNs, the primary defense cell type in the periodontal tissues. Levels of PMN-type MMPs have been shown to increase with increasing periodontal disease severity and decrease following therapy.[54] MMPs also facilitate bone resorption, by degrading unmineralized osteoid and the collagen matrix that remains after demineralization of bone by osteoclasts.

Thus, the breakdown of collagen fibers in the periodontal soft and hard tissues by MMPs, together with osteoclast-mediated bone resorption, up-regulated by pro-resorptive cytokines such as IL-1β, contributes to the clinical signs of periodontitis including pocket formation, attachment loss, bone resorption, gingival recession, tooth mobility and tooth loss.

I) Chemically Modified or Low Dose Tetracycline

The tetracyclines have been found to be effective inhibitors of matrix metalloproteinase – mediated connective tissue destruction in a variety of pathological processes. In addition to the possible effects of tetracyclines on expression, activation, and catalytic activity of matrix metalloproteinases, these compounds may have actions on other processes involved in the overall pathophysiology of multiple disease states, including regulation of release of inflammatory cytokines and glycosylation of connective tissue proteins, and they may even upregulate the expression of matrix constituents, which are produced at a deficient rate during diabetes and other diseases [R>>]. These multiple modes of action, not all of which have been sufficiently defined, may account for the positive results obtained with use of tetracyclines as therapeutic agents in models of periodontitis, as this disease process involves a complex, multifactorial pathogenesis. Other advantages during periodontal therapy are that tetracyclines[144], particularly doxycycline[145], **tend to be highly concentrated in the gingival crevicular fluid at levels 5–10 times greater than those found in serum and these antibiotics show substantivity** because they bind to the tooth structure and are slowly released as still-active agents.

All members of the tetracycline family possess the ability to down regulate MMP activity. This property was first identified in the early 1980s. Until recently, the clinical efficacy of tetracyclines such as minocycline, doxycycline and tetracycline itself has been attributed solely to their antimicrobial properties. However, **tetracyclines are now known to modulate host response.** Minocycline was further shown to inhibit PMN collagenase activity in vitro, and retard alveolar bone loss in diabetic rats. Subsequently research was focused on doxycycline, as it possesses the most potent anticollagenase properties of commercially available tetracyclines[146] Doxycyline has a much lower inhibitory concentration (IC_{50} =15 mM) than minocycline (IC_{50} =190 mM) or tetracycline (IC_{50} =350 mM), indicating that a much lower dose of doxycycline is necessary to reduce a given collagenase level by 50% compared with minocycline or tetracycline.[147] Furthermore, **doxycycline has been found to be more effective in blocking PMN-type collagenase activity (MMP-8)** than fibroblast-type collagenase activity (MMP-1) (Golub et al. 1995, Smith et al. 1999)[94,148] suggesting that doxycycline can provide a safe therapeutic method for reducing pathologically elevated collagenase levels without interfering with normal connective tissue turnover.

Doxycycline down regulates collagenolytic activity by several synergistic mechanisms. For example, doxycycline inhibits active MMPs directly by a mechanism that is dependent on its calcium- and zinc-binding properties [149]. In addition, tetracyclines are known to scavenge for, and **inhibit, the production of PMN-derived reactive oxygen metabolites,** including hypochlorous acid (H004FCl), since HOCl is known to activate latent pro-MMPs[150] and **inactivate host-derived proteinase inhibitors** (inhibitors of MMPs)[151]. Thus, the ability of tetracyclines to directly inhibit MMP activity and also scavenge for, and inhibit, reactive oxygen metabolites such as HOCl, which represents an important pathway for modulation of the destructive connective tissue events that occur in periodontitis. Moreover, **tetracyclines inhibit osteoblast and osteoclast derived MMPs,** thereby inhibiting bone resorption[152]. Doxycycline also inhibits production of epithelial cell-derived MMPs by inhibiting intracellular expression or synthesis of these enzymes[153]. Doxycyline further contributes to decreased connective tissue breakdown by down-regulating the expression of pro-inflammatory mediators such as IL-1 and TNF-α[154] and increasing collagen production, osteoblast activity and bone formation.

These and other ongoing studies on the use of this subantimicrobial low dose of doxycycline for the treatment of periodontitis have been designed to address the concerns of many in the field regarding the issue of resistance. Certain chemically modified tetracyclines have advantages over commercially-available tetracyclines because they are absorbed more rapidly, can reach higher levels in the blood, have longer serum half-lives and are more potent inhibitors of matrix metalloproteinases.

Ramamurthy et.al (2002)[100] tested the efficacy of doxycycline and 5 different chemically modified tetracyclines (CMTs) to prevent matrix metalloproteinase (MMP)-dependent periodontal tissue breakdown in an animal model of periodontitis. 96 adult male rats received intragingival injections with either 10 µl of physiologic saline or Escherkhia coli endotoxin (1 mg/ml) every other day for 6 days and were distributed into 8 treatment groups (12 rats/group): saline (S), endotoxin alone (E), E + CMT-1 , E + CMT-3, E + CMT-4, E + CMT-7, E + CMT-8, and doxycycline. All animals were treated daily with 1 ml of 2% carboxymethyl cellulose (CMC) alone or containing one of the above-mentioned CMTs (2 mg/day) orally. The gingival tissues were removed, extracted, and assayed for gelatinase (GLSE). Some rat maxillary jaws from each treatment group were fixed in buffered formalin and processed for histology and immunohistochemistry for the cytokines tumor necrosis factor (TNF), interleukin (IL)-1, and IL-6, and MMP-2 and MMP-9. Endotoxin injection induced elevated GLSE activity (functional assay and osteoclast-mediated bone resorption), the former identified as predominantly MMP-9 (92 kDa GLSE) by gelatin zymography. All 6 tetracyclines (2 mg/day) inhibited periodontal breakdown in the following order of efficacy: CMT-8 > CMT- 1 > CMT-3 > doxycycline > CMT-4 > CMT-7. Immunohistochemistry was positive for TNF, IL- 1, and IL-6 in the inflammatory cells from untreated endotoxin rat tissues, whereas treatment with CMTs decreased the number of immuno-positive stained cells for cytokines and MMPs. The authors concluded that **MMP-mediated bone loss in this model can be prevented by inhibition of MMPs using CMTs.**

Buduneli et.al (2007)[106] evaluated the individual and combined effects of low-dose doxycycline (LDD) and alendronate on gingival tissue MMP-8, -13 and -14, TIMP-1 and Ln-5 expression on endotoxin-induced periodontitis in rats. Experimental periodontitis was induced by repeated injection of LPS. Fourty-four adult male rats were divided into five study groups: saline control, LPS, LPS + doxycycline, LPS + alendronate and LPS + doxycycline + alendronate during the 7 days of the experimental study period. On day 7, the rats were sacrificed and the gingival tissues were analyzed immunohistochemically for expression of MMP-8, -13 and -14, TIMP-1 and Ln-5. Alveolar bone loss was significantly higher in the LPS, doxycycline, alendronate and combination groups than in the saline control group. Individual administration of doxycycline or alendronate significantly decreased the expression of MMP-8 compared to LPS. Combined drug administration reduced MMP-14 significantly compared to doxycycline. No significant differences in Ln-5 chain expression were found between the study groups. The authors suggested that the combined administration of doxycycline and alendronate may provide beneficial effects in periodontal treatment. They also suggested that alendronate and/or **doxycycline may inhibit MMP-8 expression significantly** and individual administration of alendronate and doxycycline results in significant increase in TIMP-1 expression in gingiva.

Golub et.al. (1995)[94] evaluated **the effect of low-dose doxycycline on host-derived collagenase activity in gingival tissues of adult periodontitis patient.** Inflamed human gingival tissue was obtained from adult periodontitis patients during periodontal surgery. The extract was then analyzed for collagenase activity using SDS-PAGE/fluorography/laser densitometry, and for gelatinase activity using type I gelatin zymography as well as a new quantitative assay using biotinylated type I gelatin as substrate. DOXY was added to the incubation mixture at a final concentration of 0-1000 µM. The concentration of DOXY required to inhibit 50% of the gingival tissue collagenase (IC_{50}) was found to be 16-18 µM in the presence or absence of 1.2 mM APMA (an optimal organomercurial activator of latent procollagenases); this IC_{50} for DOXY was similar to that exhibited for collagenase or matrix metalloproteinase (MMP)-8 from polymorphonuclear leukocytes (PMNs) and from gingival crevicular fluid (GCF) of adult periodontitis patients. Porphyromonas gingivalis collagenase was also inhibited by similar DOXY levels (IC_{50} = 15 µM). They concluded that MMPs in inflamed gingival tissue of adult periodontitis patients originate primarily from infiltrating PMNs rather than resident gingival cells or monocyte/macrophages, and that their pathologically-elevated tissue-degrading activities can be directly inhibited by pharmacologic levels of doxycycline.

Crout et.al (1996)[95] investigated the clinical results of a "cyclical" 6-month regimen of low dose doxycycline and its effect on GCF collagenase activity in adult periodontitis patients. In their double-blind, placebo-controlled study, adult periodontitis patients were administered for 6 months a "cyclical" regimen of either low dose doxycycline or placebo capsules; and various clinical parameters of periodontal disease severity, and both collagenase activity and degradation of the serum protein, $α_1$-PI, in the GCF were measured at different time periods. No significant differences between the low dose doxycycline and placebo-treated groups were observed for plaque index and gingival index. However, attachment levels, probing depth, and GCF collagenase activity and $α_1$-PI degradation were all beneficially and significantly affected by the drug regimen. The authors concluded that **low dose doxycycline inhibits tissue destruction** in the absence of either antimicrobial or significant anti-inflammatory efficacy; and that long-term low dose doxycycline could be a useful adjunct to instrumentation therapy in the management of the adult periodontitis patient.

Caton et.al (2000)[97] conducted a study which **assessed the efficacy of subantimicrobial dose doxycycline in conjunction with scaling and root planing (SRP) over a 9 month period in patients with adult periodontitis.** The effect of SDD on the dynamics of the periodontal microflora was also evaluated. 190 patients of periodontitis exhibiting clinical attachment level

[CAL] and probing depth [PD] between 5 and 9 mm including bleeding on probing [BOP] were enrolled in this double-blind, randomized, placebo-controlled, parallel-group trial. SRP was performed until the crown and root surfaces were visually and/or tactilely free of all deposits. Following SRP, patients were randomized to receive SDD 20 mg bid or placebo bid for 9 months. Patients were instructed to take study medication 1 hour before eating at approximately 12-hrs intervals. For microbial assessments, plaque samples from patients (n=76) were collected using sterile, endodontic paper points at baseline, 3, 6, and 9 months. There were significantly greater improvements in CAL and PD with adjunctive SDD than with the placebo group at 3, 6 and 9 months. The percentage of sites with AL $\geq$ 2 mm from baseline to month 9 was significantly lower with adjunctive SDD than with adjunctive placebo. Also, the percentage of patients with additional attachment loss $\geq$ 3 mm from baseline to month 9, there was a trend favoring treatment with adjunctive placebo. Reduction in PD from baseline was significantly greater for the adjunctive SDD group at every post-baseline time point than for the adjunctive placebo group. They noted improvements in clinical outcomes without detrimental shifts in the normal periodontal flora or the acquisition of doxycycline resistance or multiantibiotic resistance. They concluded that the **use of SDD 20 mg twice daily** augment the attachment gains achieved with SRP, with statistically significant **improvements in CAL and PD** relative to placebo after only 3 months of use and further improvements were evident after 6 months of SDD treatment. They did not observe a detrimental shift in the normal periodontal flora or any sort of antibiotic resistance with SDD.

Golub et.al (2001)[99] carried out a study to determine appropriate dosage of administration regimens using **subantimicrobial dose doxycycline (SDD) as an adjunctive therapy** in 75 patients with **adult periodontitis**. Primary determinants of efficacy included reductions in GCF collagenase activity and changes in relative attachment levels. Secondary efficacy parameters included changes in PD and inflammatory measurements, the latter assessed by measuring the GCF flow and the severity of gingival inflammation. The groups were as follows; Group 1- Doxycycline 20 mg bid x 12 weeks; Group 2- Doxycycline 20 mg qid x 12 weeks; Group 3- Doxycycline 20 mg bid x 4 weeks, then 20 mg qd x 8 weeks; Group 4- Doxycycline 20 mg bid x 4 weeks, then placebo x 8 weeks; Group 5- Placebo x 12 weeks. Patients were administered a scaling and prophylaxis, then 1 of 5 treatment schedules for 12 weeks (part I), followed by a 12-week period of no drug therapy (part II), a second scaling and prophylaxis, and 12 additional weeks of treatment (part III). From baseline to week 12 (part I), treatment with specially formulated SDD capsules (20 mg) twice daily for up to 12 weeks was shown to significantly reduce GCF collagenase activity and improvement in attachment levels. These effects were not seen in patients treated with placebo. Continuous drug therapy over the 12-week treatment period was needed to maintain and maximize the reduction in GCF collagenase and the improvement in attachment levels. Improvements in periodontal disease parameters occurred without the emergence of doxycycline-resistant micro-organisms. In patients administered an "on-off-on" regimen of SDD over 36 weeks (parts I-III), essentially no attachment loss occurred in patients receiving the highest of these SDD regimens (20 mg 2x daily during part I and 20 mg 1 x daily in part III), whereas patients administered placebo capsules experienced a mean attachment loss of approximately 0.8 mm at the 36-week time periods. The authors concluded that the administration of 20 mg of twice daily over an extended period can **reduce pathologic elevations in GCF collagenase activity and improve attachment level measurements** in patients with periodontitis and that the improvement in parameters occurred without any apparent side effects.

Novak et.al (2002)[101] studied the use of adjunctive host modulation therapy in form of **subantimicrobial doxycycline (SDD) for treating severe, generalized periodontitis.** Thirty subjects ≤ 45 years of age received subgingival debridement and oral hygiene instructions each week for 4 weeks, plus 6 months of adjunctive SDD or placebo. Periodontal status was monitored at baseline, and at 1, 3, 5.25, and 8.25 months following completion of the hygiene sessions. Maintenance therapy was performed at 3, 5.25, and 8.25 months for both the groups. Of the 30 subjects, the 20 subjects who completed all phases of study were equally divided into placebo and SDD group. Subgingival debridement plus adjunctive SDD reduced deep pockets (≥7 mm at baseline) by an average of 3.02 mm after 9 months versus 1.42 mm for the placebo group. A significant clinical response was seen in both groups immediately after 1 month but the response was always clinically and statistically greater in the SDD group. In the SDD group, nearly 40% of pockets ≥7 mm were reduced by ≥4 mm, and 55% were reduced by ≥3 mm. In addition, only 2 pockets deepened by ≥4 mm in the SDD group versus 10 in the placebo group. The authors concluded that full mouth **subgingival and supragingival debridement supplemented with a host modulating agent, SDD,** provides clinically and statistically significant benefits in the **reduction of deep pockets in patients with severe, generalized periodontitis.**

Emingil et.al (2004)[102] studied the **impact of Low-dose doxycycline (LDD) in combination with non-surgical periodontal therapy on gingival crevicular fluid (GCF) matrix metalloproteinase-8 (MMP-8) levels as well as on clinical parameters over a 12-month period in 30 patients with chronic periodontitis.** Every 3 months during 12 months study period GCF samples and clinical parameters including probing depth (PD), clinical attachment level (CAL), gingival index (GI), and plaque index were recorded. Patients were randomized either to receive a low-dose doxycycline or placebo group. The low-dose doxycycline group received 20 mg doxycycline bid for 3 months plus scaling and root planing (SRP), while the placebo group was given placebo capsules bid for 3 months plus SRP. GCF MMP-8 levels were determined by a time-resolved immunofluorescence assay. The low-dose doxycycline group showed a significantly greater reduction in mean PD scores at 9 and 12 months and in mean GI scores at all time points than the placebo. At 12 months CAL in low-dose doxycycline group showed greater improvement (3 mm) than the placebo group (2.2mm) but the difference was not significant. The GCF MMP-8 level in the low-dose doxycycline group was significantly lower than that of the placebo group at 6 months. The authors concluded that **adjunctive low-dose doxycycline therapy** in combination with scaling and root planing **reduces GCF MMP-8 levels and improves clinical parameters in patients with chronic periodontitis.** They also suggested that **greatest benefit of adjunctive low-dose doxycycline therapy on clinical parameters could occur about 9 months after therapy.**

Preshaw et.al (2004)[155] assessed the role of SDD (20 mg doxycycline bid) as an adjunct to scaling and root planing (SRP) in the treatment of chronic periodontitis. Two-hundred ten subjects were treated with SRP and randomly received either adjunctive SDD or placebo for 9 months. Efficacy parameters included were per-subject mean changes in clinical attachment level (CAL) and probing depth (PD) from baseline, and the total number of sites with attachment gains and probing depth reductions ≥ 2 mm and ≥ 3 mm from baseline. At sites with PD 4 to 6 mm and ≥ 7 mm (N = 209), mean improvements in CAL and PD were greater following SRP with adjunctive SDD than SRP with placebo, achieving statistical significance in all baseline disease categories at month 9. At month 9, 42.3% of sites in the SDD group demonstrated CAL gain ≥ 2 mm compared to 32.0% of sites in the placebo group. CAL gain ≥ 3 mm was seen in 15.4% of sites in the SDD group compared to 10.6% of sites in the placebo group. 42.9% of sites in the SDD group demonstrated PD reduction ≥ 2 mm as compared to 31.1% of sites in the placebo group, and 15.4% of sites in the SDD group compared to 9.1% of sites in the placebo group demonstrated PD reduction ≥ 3 mm. The authors concluded that **adjunctive SDD results in statistically significant attachment**

gains and probing depth reductions over and above those achieved by scaling and root planing with placebo.

Gurkan et.al, (2005)[104] evaluated the effect of adjunctive SDD therapy on clinical periodontal parameters and gingival crevicular fluid (GCF) transforming growth factor-beta1 (TGF-beta1) levels in patients with severe, generalized chronic periodontitis. Thirty-five patients with severe, generalized periodontitis and 11 periodontally healthy subjects were included in this clinical trial. Patients received full-mouth supragingival debridement at baseline and randomized to take either SDD bid. (n=17) or placebo bid. (n=18) for 3 months. Clinical measurements including probing depth (PD), clinical attachment level, papilla bleeding index, plaque index and GCF sampling were performed at baseline, 3 and 6 months. The GCF TGF-beta1 levels were analyzed by enzyme-linked immunosorbent assay while total $TGF-\beta_1$ was determined by using the relevant ELISA kit. Following scaling and root planing (SRP) plus SDD and SRP plus placebo therapy showed significant improvements in clinical periodontal parameters. Higher percentage of sites were reduced by at least 3 mm following adjunctive SDD therapy (66.4%) than following adjunctive placebo therapy (55.1%) at 3 months with no significant differences. However, at 6 months in the SDD group a significantly higher percentage (73.4%) of deep pockets resolved (PD reduction ≥ 3 mm from baseline) when compared with placebo group (49.7%) at 6 months. Although the mean CAL gain for sites with a baseline PD 4-6 mm and ≥ 7 mm were greater in SRP plus SDD group, when compared with SRP plus placebo group at 6 months, however, statistical analysis did not reveal significant difference. Both total amount and concentration of GCF TGF-beta1 in SDD and placebo groups were increased when compared with baseline at 3 months. The results indicated that **combination of SDD with non-surgical therapy improves clinical parameters of periodontal disease and increases GCF TGF-beta1 levels together with a decrease in prevalence.**

Preshaw et.al (2005)[105] evaluated the **role of SDD as an adjunct to scaling and root planing (SRP) in the treatment of chronic periodontitis with or without smokers** as a meta-analysis of two previously reported clinical studies. Both were 9-month, double-blind, randomized, placebo-controlled, multi-centre clinical trials that investigated the efficacy of SDD (20 mg doxycycline twice daily) in combination with SRP in subjects with moderate-severe chronic periodontitis in which 36.9% of the combined study population was smokers. 392 subjects were included in the meta-analysis, which evaluated per-subject mean changes in clinical attachment level (CAL) and probing depth (PD) from baseline and the total number of sites with attachment gains and PD reductions ≥ 2 and ≥ 3 mm from baseline in four subgroups: smokers/SDD; smokers/placebo; non-smokers/SDD; non-smokers/placebo. The authors observed a hierarchical treatment response, with non-smokers who received SDD demonstrating the greatest CAL gains and PD reductions. Smokers who received placebo demonstrated the smallest clinical improvements following treatment. Smokers who received SDD demonstrated an intermediate treatment response that was broadly equivalent to that seen in non-smokers who received placebo. They concluded that adjunctive SDD enhances therapeutic outcomes compared with SRP alone, resulting in **clinical benefit in both smokers and non-smokers with chronic periodontitis.**

Veronica and Bisada (1998)[96] compared the **efficacy of the combined systemic use of doxycycline and a non-steroidal anti-inflammatory drug (ibuprofen), either separately or in combination,** as an adjunctive treatment to scaling and root planing for adult periodontitis. Thirty-two subjects with generalized moderate adult periodontitis were randomly divided into 4 groups as follows: group 1, doxycycline 200 mg the first day followed by 100 mg per day; group 2, ibuprofen 800 mg per day; group 3, doxycycline plus ibuprofen and group 4, one placebo capsule/day (control) for 6 weeks. A split mouth design was utilized in each subject such that half of the teeth received one session of scaling and root planing (SRP), while the other half received no SRP. Plaque index (PI), gingival index (GI), probing depth and clinical attachment level (CAL) were recorded at baseline and at 3, 6, 12, and 24 weeks following SRP. At baseline there were no differences among the 4 regimens and between the SRP and without SRP groups with regard to PD and CAL. At 24 weeks, a significant reduction of mean PD was found in both doxycycline and combination group. Again, doxycycline and combination group showed significant gain of CAL from baseline. The scaling/root planing group showed significantly less PD and more CAL gain than without scaling/root planing group. The authors concluded that **systemic doxycycline alone or in combination with ibuprofen results in a statistically significant yet modest clinical improvement** in patients with moderate adult periodontitis.

Gapski et.al (2004)[103] evaluated the efficacy of access flap surgery with and without supplemental SDD for 6 months among individuals (n=24) previously unresponsive to scaling and root planing. They noted that individuals administered SDD demonstrated a statistically significantly greater probing depth reduction at sites initially more then 6 mm deep (3.3 vs 2.1 mm); however, there was no statistically significant gain of attachment level (1.8 mm vs 1.1 mm). **SDD administration also resulted in a greater reduction of levels of ICTP (a carboxyterminal fragment of type 1 collagen), which is a marker for bone resorption.**

G. Emingil (2008)[107] examined the effectiveness of a 3-month regimen of subantimicrobial dose doxycycline (SDD) in combination with scaling and root planing compared to scaling and root planing alone on levels of gingival crevicular fluid (GCF) extracellular matrix metalloproteinase inducer (EMMPRIN) in patients with chronic periodontitis. GCF samples were collected, and clinical parameters, including probing depth (PD), clinical attachment level, gingival index (GI), and plaque index, were recorded. 30 chronic periodontitis subjects were randomized to receive SDD or placebo. The

SDD group received SDD (20 mg, twice a day) for 3 months plus scaling and root planing, whereas the placebo group took placebo capsules twice a day for 3 months and received scaling and root planing. The subjects were reevaluated at 3 and 6 months. At each visit, all clinical parameters were measured and GCF was sampled. GCF EMMPRIN levels were determined by Western immunoblotting assay. Results were in favor of SDD & a significant improvement was observed in all clinical parameters in the SDD group over the 6-month study period. The SDD group showed a significantly greater reduction in mean PD scores at 6 months and in mean GI scores at 3 and 6 months than the placebo group. From baseline to 6 months, the GCF EMMPRIN levels were reduced significantly in the SDD group. The GCF EMMPRIN level in the SDD group was significantly lower than that of the placebo group at 3 and 6 months. The authors concluded that SDD therapy in combination with scaling and root planing reduced GCF EMMPRIN levels and improved clinical periodontal parameters in subjects with chronic periodontitis. The ability of **SDD to downregulate, in vivo, the GCF levels of EMMPRIN,** a unique upregulator of matrix metalloproteinase expression, is one of its beneficial host-modulatory properties.

Golub.M et al (2008)[108] tested the hypothesis of **subantimicrobial-dose doxycycline modulating gingival crevicular fluid biomarkers of periodontitis in postmenopausal (PM) osteopenic women.** GCF was collected from SDD- and placebo-treated PM subjects (n = 64 each) at the baseline and 1- and 2-year appointments; the volume was determined; and the samples were analyzed for collagenase activity (using a synthetic peptide as substrate), relative levels of three genetically distinct collagenases (Western blot), a type-1 collagen breakdown product/bone resorption marker (a carboxyterminal telopeptide cross-link fragment of type I collagen [ICTP]; radioimmunoassay), and interleukin-1β (enzyme-linked immunosorbent assay). Collagenase activity was significantly reduced by SDD treatment relative to placebo. ICTP showed a similar pattern of change during SDD treatment, and GCF collagenase activity and ICTP were positively correlated at all time periods. Matrix metalloproteinase (MMP)-8 accounted for ~80% of total collagenase in GCF, with much less MMP-1 and -13. Thus, the observations of the study support the **therapeutic potential of long-term SDD therapy to reduce periodontal collagen breakdown and alveolar bone resorption in PM women.**

All the above results corroborate the beneficial use of CMT in treatment of periodontal disease & recent results have expanded the usefulness of SDD therapy as an adjunct to scaling and root planing in the long-term management of periodontal disease.

II) Bisphosphonate Therapy

Most recently bisphosphonates, primarily designed to modulate osteoclast function and not specifically designed to be matrix metalloproteinase inhbitors, have been found to inhibit matrix metalloproteinases 1, 3, 8 and 13 (Teronen O, 1997)[234] by cation chelation mechanism. Biophosphates are one host-modulating class of drugs that has demonstrated this ability. These drugs are clinically effective at reducing bone resorption and have shown the ability to inhibit host degradative enzymes, specifically the matrix metalloproteinases (MMPs).

H. Nakaya et al (2000)[98] investigated the **regulatory effects of a bisphosphonate, tiludronate, on MMP levels and activity in human periodontal cells.** MMP-1 and MMP-3 were assessed in cultured human periodontal ligament cells treated with a bisphosphonate, tiludronate. Reverse transcription-polymerase chain reaction (RT-PCR) was used to identify mRNA levels for both enzymes, and also for tissue inhibitors (TIMP-1). Enzyme immunoassay (EIA) and immunocytochemistry were used to assess MMP proteins in these cell cultures. Enzyme activity was assessed using

FITCconjugated substrates and quantitated using spectrophotofluorometry. Results of the study showed that Tiludronate significantly inhibited both MMP-1 and MMP-3 activity in a concentration-dependent manner. A maximal reduction in activity of 35% was achieved for each of the enzymes at a 10^{-4} M concentration. Tiludronate did not have a significant effect on the mRNA levels for MMP-1, MMP-3, or TIMP-1. Similarly, there were no effects noted for either MMP-1 or MMP-3 on the protein level. **This study demonstrates an inhibitory effect of tiludronate on the activity of both MMP-1 and MMP-3.** These effects appear to occur without altering either mRNA or protein levels for these enzymes, supporting a possible mechanism of action that involves the ability of bisphosphonates to chelate cations from the MMPs.

Buduneli et.al (2007)[106] evaluated the individual and combined effects of low-dose doxycycline (LDD) and alendronate on gingival tissue MMP-8, -13 and -14, TIMP-1 and Ln-5 expression on endotoxin-induced periodontitis in rats. The authors suggested that the combined administration of doxycycline and alendronate may provide beneficial effects in periodontal treatment. They also suggested that **alendronate and/or doxycycline may inhibit MMP-8 expression significantly and individual administration of alendronate and doxycycline results in significant increase in TIMP-1 expression in gingiva.**

All these corroborate that Bisphosphonates have a potential to modulate MMPs & these results support the continued investigation of these drugs as potential therapeutic agents in periodontal disease

III) Synthetic Inhibitors of Metalloproteinases

Zn^{2+} and Ca^{2+}-chelating agents (EDTA and 1, 10- phenanthroline) are potent inhibitors of enzyme activity *in vitro*, but they are toxic and not used *in vivo* as therapeutic agents (Greenwald R., 1995)[85]. Multiple synthetic peptides have been formulated in an attempt to synthesize more specific chelators including phosphorus containing peptides, sulfur-based inhibitors and peptidyl hydroxamic acid derivatives. Phosphorus containing peptides are potent inhibitors of metalloproteinases produced by the substitution of a tetrahedral phosphorus atom for the carbonyl carbon atom in a peptide substrate. Phosphonamidate and phosphinate analogs of tripeptides have been shown to inhibit human skin fibroblast collagenase *in vitro* (Galardy R, 1992).[157] Sulfur based inhibitors of the matrix metalloproteinases were prepared by replacing the scissile C (=0)-NH bond of the peptide with various sulfur-containing functional groups. The mercaptan derivatives were the most potent inhibitors of collagenases, gelatinases and stromelysin compared with all other sulfur based inhibitors of matrix metalloproteinases *in vitro* (Schwartz M, 1992).[158] Perhaps the most widely used synthetic peptides, and the ones receiving the most attention as potential pharmaceutical agents, are the hydroxamic acid derivatives. These are prepared by adding a hydroxamic acid residue at the C-terminus of the peptide as a metal-chelating moiety (Nagai Y, 1992).[159] Hydroxamic acid derivatives have been shown to inhibit matrix metalloproteinases 1, 2, 3, 7, 8 and 9 *in vitro* with very low levels at which collagenase activity declines by 50% (such as the low nM range) (Nagai Y, 1992).[159]

Modulation of host response with SDD as an adjunct to mechanical debridement has scientific merit, and there appear to be no adverse side effects. The clinically significant benefits of subantimicrobial dose doxycycline when used in addition to high quality SRP are apparent. SDD in combination with mechanical procedures has been shown to be effective in improving probing depths and attachment levels compared with mechanical debridement alone. **No antimicrobial effect was detected during or following a 9 month treatment regimen with 20 mg SDD bid on total bacterial count, the normal flora, or in either periodontal or opportunistic pathogens.** Several clinical trials administered SDD for 9 months. Caton et.al[97] achieved 90 % of their final clinical results within 3 months. This seems reasonable, as others indicated that

SDD need to be administered for 12 consecutive weeks to maximally lower collagenase levels (Golub, 2001).[99] The duration for which adjunctive SDD needs to be administered to obtain optimal results is not clear. It appears that **3 months of adjunctive SDD achieves most of the therapy's potential benefits in patients with chronic periodontitis.** However, prolonged use (eg, 9 months) may further improve the results.

Apart from SDD various synthetic inhibitors have also been tried. The most widely used and potent of these are the mercaptan derivatives and the Hydroxamic acid derivatives. Both haven been shown to inhibit the matrix metalloproteinases in vitro. Bisphosphonates, used primarily for modulation of bone remodeling have also been shown to inhibit matrix metalloproteinases.

C) <u>MODULATION OF HOST CYTOKINES</u>

Cytokines are defined as regulatory proteins controlling the survival, growth, differentiation and functions of cells. Cytokines are produced transiently at generally low concentrations, act and are degraded in a local environment. The pro-inflammatory cytokines like Interleukins (IL) and tumor necrosis factor (TNF) have been implicated in the progression of periodontal disease. Based upon the increased expression of IL-1 and TNF in inflamed gingiva and high levels in the GCF of periodontitis patients, several studies have suggested that increased production of these cytokines may play an important role in periodontal tissue destruction.[10] To prevent an uncontrolled inflammatory response with rapid tissue destruction, the activities of IL-1 and TNF-α are naturally counteracted by the production of cytokines such as IL-4, IL-10 and IL-11.[65]

Soluble Cytokine Antagonists

Blocking the activity of pro-inflammatory cytokines may be a beneficial therapeutic modality for periodontitis. To counteract tissue destruction and maintain homeostasis, cytokine antagonists such as IL-1 receptor antagonist (IL-1Ra) or soluble TNF receptors have been shown to inhibit competitively receptor-mediated signal transduction.[58]

Assuma et al. (1998)[109] investigated the **effects of function-blocking soluble receptors to IL-1 and TNF** applied by local injection at sites with induced periodontal destruction and compared with similar sites injected with vehicle alone during ligature-induced experimental periodontitis in Monkey model. Activity of IL-1 and TNF were inhibited by soluble receptors to pro-inflammatory cytokines via local injection into interdental papillae. The results indicated that injection of soluble receptors to IL-1 and TNF inhibited by approximately 80% the recruitment of inflammatory cells in close proximity to bone. The **formation of osteoclasts was reduced by 67%** at the experimental sites compared with that at the control sites, and the amount of bone loss was reduced by 60%.

Graves et.al (1998)[110] investigated the role of interleukin-1 (IL-1) as well as tumor necrosis factor (TNF) in the temporal movement of inflammatory cells toward the alveolar bone and the effect of topical application of soluble receptors to IL-1 and TNF in this process in a Macaca fascicularis primate model of experimental periodontitis. IL-1 and TNF activity was inhibited by local application of soluble receptors to IL-1 and TNF by injection into interdental papillae. The results indicated that following induction of experimental periodontitis, the front of inflammatory cells progressed toward alveolar bone and was associated with osteoclast formation. These processes were inhibited by blockers to IL-1 and TNF. The authors concluded that local injection of **soluble receptors to IL-1 and TNF inhibited osteoclast**

formation and progression of inflammatory cell infiltration towards alveolar bone.

Oates et.al (2002)[114] assessed clinical, radiographic, and biochemical markers as diagnostic indicators of disease activity by comparing ligature-induced bone loss in the presence or absence of IL-1/TNF-α antagonist inhibition of bone loss in a primate model. Six animals with a naturally-occurring gingivitis were evaluated over a 6-week time period following the placement of silk ligatures and initiation of a soft diet. Three animals received intra-papillary injections of soluble receptors (blockers), capable of blocking the biologic activity of both IL-1 and TNF-α, and 3 animals received vehicle (control) injections. Injections were given 3 times per week over the course of the study. Clinical assessments included a gingival index and quantification of gingival crevicular fluid (GCF) levels. Collected GCF samples were then used for the biochemical assessment of pyridinoline (PYD) and bone alkaline phosphatase (BAP). Radiographic assessment was made using computer-assisted subtraction radiography to measure both bone density (CADIA) values and linear changes in crestal bone height. The use of the blockers significantly (p, 0.01) reduced the levels of radiographic bone loss by approximately 50% compared with that of the control sites. Both biochemical markers showed the greatest increase during the first two weeks of the study with PYD levels increased 35-fold over baseline levels after 1 week. This difference in response was significantly (p, 0.05) greater than the levels found in the non-ligated teeth or in the ligated teeth receiving blockers injections. BAP levels showed significant increase in ligated teeth compared to non-ligated teeth, but failed to show any significant difference between animals treated with vehicle and those treated with IL-1/TNF antagonists. No significant differences in GI, and GCF amounts were observed comparing the experimental group with the placebo group.

Delima (2001)[113] investigated the role of IL-1 and TNF in the loss of connective tissue attachment and the effect of topical application of soluble receptors to these cytokines on preventing loss of connective tissue attachment, thereby preventing progression of periodontitis in a Macaca fascicularis primate model of experimental periodontitis. Silk ligatures impregnated with the periodontal pathogen, Porphyromonas gingivalis were wrapped around the posterior teeth and the activity of IL-1 and TNF were found to be inhibited by soluble receptors to these proinflammatory cytokines via local injection into interdental papillae. Histomorphometric analysis indicated that IL-1 and TNF antagonists significantly reduced the loss of connective tissue attachment by approximately 51% and the loss of alveolar bone height by almost 91%. The authors concluded that the **loss of connective tissue attachment and progression of periodontal disease can be retarded by antagonists to specific host mediators such as IL-1 and TNF.**

Martuscelli et al. (2000)[112] studied the effects of recombinant human IL-11 (rhIL-11) by subcutaneous administration to prevent progression of attachment loss and radiographic bone loss in a ligature induced beagle dog model. Twenty female dogs were divided into three treatment groups and one control group. The three treatment groups received subcutaneous injections of 15, 30, or 80 µg/kg of rhIL-11 in saline buffer twice a week. The placebo received buffer only twice a week. Presence or absence of gingival inflammation, plaque and bleeding on probing were recorded. Attachment levels and bone height were also measured. At week 8, the placebo group had 3.89 mm of attachment loss and 73.8 % radiographic bone remaining. The group receiving 15 µg/kg of rhIL-11 showed 1.99 mm of attachment loss and 89.5 % radiographic bone remaining; the group receiving 30 µg/kg of rhIL-11 showed 0.84 mm of attachment loss and 92.5 % radiographic bone remaining while the group receiving 80 µg/kg of rhIL-11 showed 1.05 mm of attachment loss and 85.5 % bone remaining. All three treatment groups lost significantly less attachment and retained significantly more bone than did the placebo group. The authors concluded that the subcutaneous injections of rhIL-11 can inhibit the progression of attachment loss and radiographic bone loss in experimental periodontitis model.

In diabetics, the chronically elevated glucose levels result in an accelerated formation of advanced glycation end-products (AGEs). AGEs represent a heterogeneous class of non-enzymatically glycated proteins and lipids found in plasma, vessel walls and tissues. Endothelial cells and monocytes possess specific receptors for AGEs called RAGEs located on their cell surfaces.[160] Studies have shown that the interaction of AGEs with their receptors (RAGEs) plays an important role in the development of diabetic complications.[161] The interaction of macrophages with AGEs has been shown to stimulate increased secretions of cytokines such as TNF-α and IL-1.[162] In diabetic mice, blockade of RAGEs with soluble receptors (sRAGEs) suppressed periodontitis associated bone loss and reduced the levels of IL-6, TNF- α and MMPs.[163]

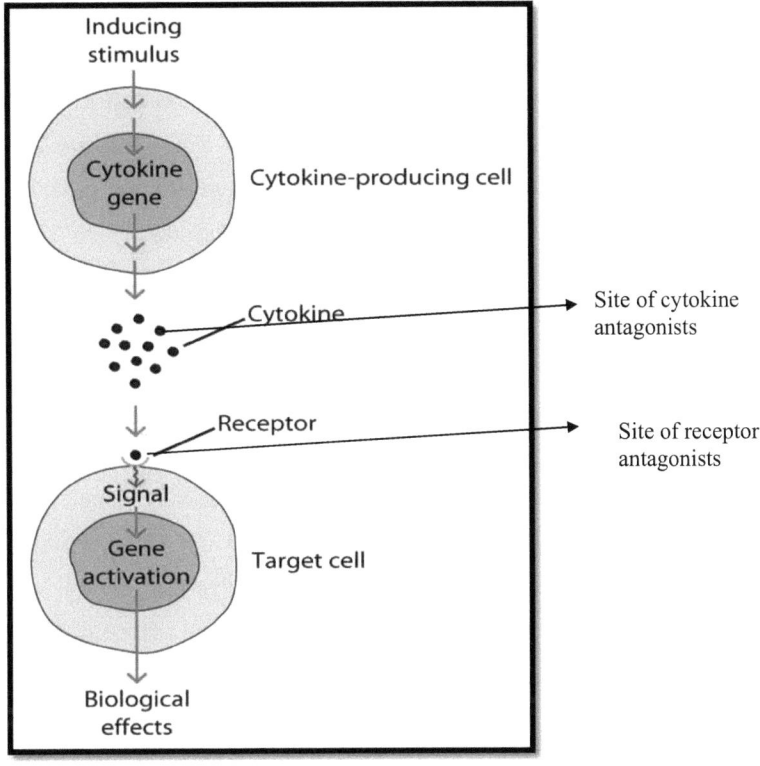

Fig.7. Picture showing sites o action of soluble cytokine antagonists.

Investigations on the soluble protein delivery of antagonists to interleukin-1 and tumor necrosis factor in a primate model of periodontitis have shown promising results. Collectively, the clinical, radiographic and biochemical findings of these experiments showed that IL-1 and TNF-α antagonists blocked the progression of the inflammatory cell infiltrate towards the alveolar crest, the recruitment of osteoclasts and prevent the loss of periodontal attachment and alveolar bone. Further, the findings of **Martuscelli et al. (2000)**[112] indicated that subcutaneous injection of recombinant human IL-11 (rhIL-11) was able to alter periodontal disease progression measured by changes in attachment level and radiographic bone height. However, a harsh enzymatic environment in periodontal lesions may destroy the soluble cytokine antagonists prior to their peak activity, which may necessitate more frequent administration of the active agents to the defects. Thus, gene transfer of TNFr antagonists and IL-1r antagonists may offer a more efficient mode of delivery of disease controlling agents to the periodontal structures.

Cytokines function as a network, are produced by different cell types and share overlapping features. While very few biological responses are mediated by only one cytokine, many responses can be achieved by several different cytokines. Thus, important cellular functions are usually backed up in mechanisms, where one cytokine can compensate for the loss of another. Consequently, blocking one inflammatory mediator or cytokine will not assure that a receptor-mediated response will not be activated by alternate pathways. This would require the development of polypharmaceutical approaches controlling all pathways associated with inflammation and tissue destruction.

D) MODULATION OF NITRIC OXIDE SYNTHASE (NOS) ACTIVITY

Nitric oxide (NO) is a short-lived molecule implicated in a wide range of biological processes. NO is formed by the oxidation of L-arginine through the different nitric oxide synthase (NOS). NOS are produced physiologically in endothelium, central and peripheral nerves and are classified as endothelial NOS (eNOS) and neuronal NOS (nNOS), whereas inducible form of NOS (iNOS) is expressed in response to pro-inflammatory stimuli. eNOS and nNOS are named as constitutive NOS (cNOS) and produce modest levels of NO for a short period. Conversely, iNOS forms large amount of NO for a longer period (Nathan C, 1997)[14] and is expressed by epithelial cells, fibroblast cells, and inflammatory cells in response to proinflammatory mediators, such as IL-1β, TNF-α and interferon-γ [164] and bacterial LPS. However, endogenous cytokines such as transforming growth factor β (TGF- β), IL-4 and IL-10 decreases iNOS expression in macrophages. [165]

It has been suggested that the overproduction of NO by iNOS during inflammation may be related to tissue destruction. Nitric oxide synthase (NOS) inhibitors have demonstrated protective effects against bone resorption and inflammatory process in ligature-induced periodontitis in rats.[111] Although NO has an antimicrobial protective activity, its elevated concentration in the tissues has a cytotoxic effect toward the host cell.

Inhibitors of NO (MEG, PARP)

Animal experiments have shown that pharmacological inhibition of iNOS with mercaptoalkylguanidines was associated with decreased inflammation, haemorrhagic shock and arthritis scores.[166] This may be explained by the fact that this class of drugs (e.g. mercaptoethylguanidines (MEGs)) is able to (i) inhibit COX [166], (ii) scavenge peroxinitrite [167] and (iii) block iNOS.[167]

Lohinai et.al, (1998)[111] investigated the potential protective effect of mercaptoethylguanidine (MEG) on the bone loss associated with periodontitis in ligature induced periodontitis in 30 Wistar rats. Animals were divided into two groups (15 rats each): one group of rats was treated with MEG 30 mg/ kg, i.p., 4 times per day for 8 days, animals in the other group received vehicle. At day 8, the gingivomucosal tissue encircling the mandibular 1st molars was removed on both sides for inducible nitric oxide synthase (iNOS) activity assay and for immunocytochemistry with anti-iNOS serum. Plasma extravasation was measured with the Evans blue technique. Alveolar bone loss was measured with a videomicroscopy. Ligation caused a significant; more than 3 fold increase in the gingival iNOS activity, whereas it did not affect iNOS activity on the contralateral side. The authors reported that **ligature-induced**

periodontitis showed increase in local NO production and that MEG treatment protects against the associated extravasation and bone destruction.

Recently, the role of activation and pharmacological inhibition of nuclear poly (ADP-ribose) polymerase (PARP) enzyme, a mediator of downstream NO toxicity, was investigated using the ligature- induced periodontitis model in rats and mice. **Lohinai et al. (2003)**[115] investigated the role of the activation of nuclear poly (ADP-ribose) polymerase (PARP) enzyme, a mediator of downstream nitric oxide toxicity, using a combined approach of pharmacological inhibition and genetic disruption in a ligature-induced-periodontitis model in rats and mice. After ligature placement around the neck of the first left mandibular molar, the rats were administered a potent PARP inhibitor (e.g. PJ34) or vehicle by intraperitoneal injection. Non-ligated right first mandibular molars served as controls. Immunohistochemical analysis revealed significantly increased poly (ADP-ribose) nuclear staining (indicative of PARP activation) in the subepithelial connective tissue of the ligated side compared with the non-ligated side. Ligation-induced periodontitis resulted in marked plasma extravasation in the gingivomucosal tissue and led to alveolar bone destruction compared with the non-ligated side, as measured by the Evans blue technique and by videomicroscopy, respectively. PARP inhibition with PJ34, as well as genetic PARP-1 deficiency, significantly reduced the extravasation and the alveolar bone resorption of the ligated side compared with controls. Thus, **PARP activation contributes to the development of periodontal injury. Inhibition of PARP may represent a novel host response modulatory approach for the therapy of periodontitis.**

In conclusion, in animal experimental periodontitis, the use of pharmacological inhibitors of NO and PARP synthases may reduce periodontal attachment and bone loss.

The use of selective iNOS inhibitors, mercaptoalkylguanidines has been demonstrated to reduce loss of periodontal attachment and bone in animal experimental periodontitis. Further, the use of pharmacological inhibitors of NO and PARP synthase also have been shown to reduce loss of periodontal attachment and bone. However, further studies are necessary to determine the applicability of these agents as therapeutic drugs. It is conceived that new potential agents to modulate host response may be developed in future.

E) ENAMEL MATRIX PROTEIN AS A HOST MODULATING AGENT

An ideal goal of periodontal treatment is periodontal regeneration. Several products have been developed & used in clinical practice with variable results. One of these is enamel matrix derivative which consists of hydrophobic enamel matrix proteins extracted from porcine developing enamel. Many investigators have reported that use of enamel matrix proteins improves clinical periodontal attachment without evidence of local & systemic inflammatory events. [168] There are many local host modulation agents that have been investigated but only host modulation agent currently **approved by FDA** for adjunctive use during surgery is enamel matrix proteins (Emdogain).

Mohamed H. Parkar et al (2004)[127] conducted a study to explore the selective effects of EMD on the activities of 268 cytokine, growth factor, and receptor genes in PDL. PDL cells were cultured in the absence and presence of EMD at a concentration of 100 µg/ml for 4 days. RNA was extracted and used to generate labeled cDNA probes. These were hybridized to cDNA arrays comprising 268 genes and exposed to x-ray films. Autoradiographs were digitized and analyzed. 46 percent (125 of 268) of the tested genes were found to be expressed by the PDL cells. Of these 125 genes, 38 were differentially expressed by PDL cells which had been cultured in the presence of EMD. Among the 38, 12 were found to be downregulated, notably mostly inflammatory genes, whereas 26 genes demonstrated upregulation, many of these coding for growth factors and growth factor receptors. The present study has shown that **EMD downregulates the expression of genes involved in the early inflammatory phases of wound healing while simultaneously upregulating genes encoding growth and repair-promoting molecules.** This may partly explain the apparent efficacy of EMD application in periodontal regeneration.

Sunao Sato et al (2008)[133] conducted a study which was aimed at **evaluating the influence of EMD on inflammatory-associated markers using an in vitro monocyte assay.** Rat monocytes were exposed to lipopolysaccharide (LPS; 100 ng/ml from *Escherichia coli* or *Actinobacillus actinomycetemcomitans*) along with EMD (0, 50, 100, or 200 µg/ml). Levels of tumor necrosis factor-alpha (TNF-α) and prostaglandin E_2 (PGE_2) in conditioned media were analyzed by enzyme-linked immunosorbent assay. In addition, the effects of exogenous PGE_2 on TNF-α production from LPS-stimulated monocytes were determined. Results of this study showed that LPS-stimulated monocytes exposed to EMD exhibited a decrease in TNF-α production (0.10- to 0.52-fold) and an increase in PGE_2 production (1.31- to 2.71-fold) compared to controls not treated with EMD. Exogenously applied PGE_2 decreased TNF-α production by LPS-stimulated monocytes in a dose-dependent manner, and EMD treatment enhanced this PGE_2-mediated inhibition of TNF-α production. This study concluded that **EMD modulates two inflammation-associated factors, TNF-α and PGE_2, in monocytes.**

Thus all these data suggest that in addition to enamel matrix proteins published role in inducing proliferation, migration, adhesion, mineralization, and differentiation of periodontal ligament cells, enamel matrix protein also have a potential anti-inflammatory effect.

F) MODULATION OF BONE REMODELING

The discovery of a novel receptor called osteoprotegerin (OPG) revealed a key regulatory mechanism in osteoclast differentiation and activity. Briefly, OPG (RANK) and receptor activator of NF-k B ligand (RANKL) are two molecules that regulate osteoclast formation and bone resorption. RANKL induces osteoclast differentiation and activation, whereas OPG (RANK) blocks this process by acting as a decoy receptor for RANKL. RANKL mediates a signal for osteoclastogenesis through RANK on pre-osteoclast cells. In summary, the RANKL/RANK interaction is responsible for differentiation and maturation of osteoclast precursor cells to activate osteoclasts. Osteoprotegerin acts as a decoy receptor, expressed by osteoblastic cells, which binds to RANKL and inhibits osteoclast development. Several studies have shown the opposite effect of RANKL and osteoprotegerin in bone modulation. Moreover, several stimulators of bone resorption that up-regulate RANKL expression inhibit osteoprotegerin expression in osteoblast stromal cells.[63]

Factors regulating osteoblast and osteoclast activity have become targets for developing pharmacological and clinical strategies to modulate the rate of bone formation and resorption. Targeting the host modulation via inhibition of bone resorption may be accomplished by altering differentiation of osteoclast, the specific component necessary for the process of resorption, or the duration of their activity via reducing their lifespan.

I) Osteoprotegerin (OPG)

The use of osteoprotegerin as a therapeutic agent was first evaluated by Simonet et al.[169] when they treated ovariectomized rats with murine osteoprotegerin-Fe protein and protected them against losses of bone volume associated with deficiencies of estrogen. Other preclinical studies demonstrated a potential therapeutic role of osteoprotegerin in the prevention and reduction of lytic bone lesions associated with skeletal tumor, prostatic carcinoma metastases, hypercalcemia of malignancy and breast cancer.

The use of osteoprotegerin as an inhibitor of bone alveolar destruction in periodontal disease was investigated in mice orally infected with A. a comitans (Mahamed DA, 2005).[170] Inhibition of RANKL function with osteoprotegerin treatment significantly reduced the number of osteoclasts and the alveolar bone destruction in both studies.

Qiming Jin et al (2007)[132] evaluated the effect of osteoprotegrin (OPG) on RANKL inhibition & its effects on alveolar bone resorption. An experimental ligature-induced model of periodontitis was used for the study. A total of 32 rats were administered human OPG-Fc fusion protein (10 mg/kg) or vehicle by subcutaneous delivery twice weekly for 6 weeks. Negative or positive controls received no treatment or disease through vehicle delivery, respectively. Biopsies were harvested after 3 and 6 weeks, and mandibulae were evaluated by microcomputed tomography (μCT) and histology. Serum levels of human OPG-Fc and tartrate-resistant acid phosphatase-5b (TRAP-5b) were measured throughout the study by enzyme-linked immunosorbent assay (ELISA). Human OPG-Fc was detected in the sera of OPG-Fc–treated animals by 3 days and throughout the study. Results of the study showed that serum TRAP-5b was sharply decreased by OPG-Fc treatment soon after OPG-Fc delivery and remained low for the observation period. Significant preservation of alveolar bone volume was observed among OPG-Fc–treated animals compared to the controls at weeks 3 and 6. Descriptive histology revealed that OPG-Fc significantly suppressed osteoclast surface area at the alveolar crest. The authors concluded that **systemic delivery of OPG-Fc inhibits alveolar bone resorption in experimental periodontitis,** suggesting that RANKL inhibition may represent an important therapeutic strategy for the prevention of progressive alveolar bone loss.

II) Bisphosphonates

Another approach is modulation of bone remodelling with the use of bisphosphonates. Bisphosphonates represent a class of chemical compounds structurally related to pyrophosphate, a natural product of human metabolism present in the serum and urine with calcium-chelating properties.[105] Pyrophosphate regulates mineralization by binding to hydroxyapatite crystals in vitro but it is not stable in vivo, undergoing rapid hydrolysis of its labile P–O–P bond as a result of phyrophosphatase activity. The replacement of the linking oxygen atom with a carbon atom (e.g. P–C–P) results in the formation of a bisphosphonate molecule. This compound is chemically stable and completely resistant to enzymatic hydrolysis via pyrophosphatase and alkaline phosphatase. Thus, bisphosphonate have an affinity to bind to hydroxyapatite crystals and prevent their growth and dissolution and they have an ability to increase osteoblast differentiation and inhibit osteoclast recruitment and activity, hence they are widely used in the management of systemic metabolic bone disorders such as tumour-induced hypercalcaemia, osteoporosis and Paget's disease.[172]

In the management of periodontal disease-associated bone loss, administration of bisphosphonates may have potential applications. Findings from in vitro experiments demonstrated that bisphosphonates down-regulated activity levels of several MMPs (Teronen et al. 1999).[156]

Brunsvold et.al (1992)[116] determined the effect of a bisphosphonate compound on the development of periodontitis using the non-human primate model. 27 adult cynomolgus monkeys were included in the study. Baseline data included including plaque index, gingival index, clinical probing depth measurements, and intraoral radiographs. Standardized radiographs were analyzed for quantitative changes in bone density using a computer assisted densitometric (CADIA) system. Animals were divided into 3 groups to receive 1 of the 3 treatment agents; these agents consisted of two levels of the test drug (alendronate) and a saline placebo. Concentrations of the test drug were 0.05 mg/Kg and 0.25 mg/Kg. Agents were injected in the saphenous vein of the lower leg every 2 weeks for 16 weeks. One week after the initiation of treatment agent injections, mandibular right molars and premolars were ligated with 3-0 silk sutures to induce periodontitis. Ligated teeth were inoculated with Porphyromonas gingivalis to insure a significant etiologic challenge. Nonligated homologous teeth served as controls. Clinical measurements and radiographs were repeated at 8 and 16 weeks after ligation. The test drug in both concentrations had a little effect on probing depths, gingival index or plaque compared to control animals. The bisphosphonate at a concentration of 0.05 mg/kg produced less density loss than either the placebo or 0.25 groups. The higher level dose of the test drug did not differ from placebo with respect to loss of bone density. The authors concluded that alendronate, a **bisphosphonate, significantly inhibited bone density loss** in periodontitis without significantly affecting the plaque index, gingival index or probing depth measurements.

Reddy (1995)[173] evaluated the **effect of the bisphosphonate drug alendronate on radiographic bone loss and clinical parameters** associated with the progression of periodontitis in the naturally occurring beagle dog model. Sixteen 7 to 9 year old beagles with moderate-to-severe periodontitis were studied for 6 months. Clinical measurements of attachment level, gingival index, plaque index, and mobility were performed monthly. Intraoral radiographs were made at baseline and at 3 and 6 months. The radiographs were analyzed by digital image analysis of the subtracted radiographs. At month 6 the animals were sacrificed and examined by histomorphometric analysis. The dogs were stratified into two groups based on initial periodontal severity. One group received 3.0 mg/kg alendronate weekly orally and the other group received a placebo. Silk ligatures were placed on the study teeth for the first 3 months of the study to exacerbate the periodontal destruction. The mandibles were processed for histolology at month 6. A trend toward decreased attachment loss and mobility was observed in favor of the alendronate group. A significant difference in bone density was found by histomorphometric analysis whereas no effect on the clinical parameters of gingival inflammation or plaque. . Overall, the alendronate group lost 0.2 ±0.1mm and the placebo group 1.4±0.1 mm of bone height during the 6 month study. The authors concluded that the administration of **bisphosphonate reduces bone loss associated with periodontitis progression** and the may provide a strong adjunctive effect in the management adult periodontal patients.

Yaffe et.al (1995)[118] tested the ability of amino hydroxybutylidene bisphosphonate (AB) to suppress alveolar bone loss during the initial phase of regional accelerated phenomenon following mucoperiosteal flap surgery and also compared local application and systemic administration of different concentrations of AB. 63 Wistar male rats were used in this experiment. They were divided as follows: group A, 15 rats received 0.05 mg/kg body weight of AB; group B, 15 rats received 0.25 mg/kg body weight of AB; group C, 15 rats received 0.5 mg/kg body weight of AB; group D control (18) received injection of saline. The AB or saline in the control group was administered one week prior to surgery, at the day of surgery and one week following the surgery. The drug was administered IV in the dorsal vein of the penis. The mucoperiosteal flap surgery was performed both on the buccal and lingual aspects in the region of premolars and molars of the right side of the mandible, one quadrant per rat. In another set of experiments AB was locally applied at 3 dose levels using a wet gauze sponge soaked with a solution of 0.15, 0.75, and 1.5 mg/ml on the exposed bone in the experimental side, and saline on the exposed bone on the control side for 10 seconds. The rats were sacrificed 3 weeks following the flap procedure. High resolution x-ray microradiographic analysis of 1 to 1.5 mm thick ground sections between premolar and molar region of the mandible in a buccal-lingual direction (4 to 5 sections in each side of the mandible) was performed. In one group of rats, in which AB was applied locally for 10 seconds directly onto the exposed alveolar bone during surgery in 3 concentrations (0.15, 0.75, and 1.5 mg/ml) had no noticeable effect on reducing bone resorption. In another series of experiments, in which AB was administered systemically (IV), using concentrations of 0.05, 0.25, and 0.5 mg/kg body weight showed reduced alveolar bone resorption. The rats that received 0.05 mg/kg body weight of AB revealed large areas of radiolucency which correlate to massive resorption of alveolar bone. The group that received 0.25 mg/kg body weight of AB showed reduced areas of radiolucency. The group administered with 0.5 mg/kg body weight of AB demonstrated marked reduction of bone resorption. The authors suggested **prescribing the AB for patients before periodontal or implant surgery, and following surgery is beneficial to prevent or minimize bone resorption.**

Yaffe et.al (1997)[120] evaluated the **effect of local delivery of the amino bisphosphonate on bone resorption as an adjuvant to mucoperiosteal flaps.** 25 Wistar rats were used in this experiment. The right side of the mandible served as the experimental side {amino bisphosphonate [AB]} while the left side as a control (saline). Following mucoperiosteal flap elevation in the premolar and molar region of the rat mandible, a surgical pellet soaked with 0.025 ml of amino bisphosphonate was locally applied on the exposed bone surface and covered by flap in the experimental side (right, AB). Rats were sacrificed 21 days following the flap procedure. High resolution x-ray microradiography analysis was performed. The ground sections were performed between the premolar and molar region of the mandible in a buccal-lingual direction (4 or 5 sections in each side of the mandible). Large areas of extensive bone resorption resulting in alveolar bone loss were observed in cross sections at 3 weeks after mucoperiosteal flap surgery. Topical application of the pellet soaked in 0.025 ml of the AB solution (20 mg/ml) demonstrated marked reduction of bone resorption, maintaining the height of the alveolar crest. The mean bone surface in the topically treated side (AB) was 18.96 ± 1.37 mm² compared to the contralateral side of the mandible, (saline) 12.50 ± 0.57. Topical application of the amino bisphosphonate showed reduces loss of alveolar bone by 52%. This reduced bone loss was highly significant. **Image processing analysis showed higher bone density at the AB-treated sites in comparison to saline sites.** The authors concluded that local application of amino bisphosphonate could be used as an adjunct in therapy for reducing bone resorption following surgery

Weinreb et.al (1994)[117] tested the efficacy of alendronate, a bisphosphonate, in reducing alveolar bone loss caused by experimental periodontitis in monkeys. Ligature induced periodontitis was developed in mandibular molars along with inoculation of P. gingivalis. Contralateral, homologous non-ligated teeth served as controls. Animals received, intravenously, either saline or alendronate at 0.05 or 0.25 mg/kg every 2 weeks for 16 weeks. After the animals were sacrificed, histomorphometrical analysis was done. There were no side effects seen in any of the animals. In saline treated animals, ligation and inoculation resulted in significant bone loss both at CEJ and at furcation. Alendronate at 0.05 mg/kg had significantly reduced bone loss at both sites. In contrast the 0.25 mg/kg was ineffective in attenuating alveolar bone loss in furcation area and was only slightly effective in preventing it at CEJ area. **The authors concluded that alendronate could reduce the loss of alveolar bone support associated with periodontitis.**

Shoji et.al (1995)[119] examined the **effect of systemic administration of a bisphosphonate, risedronate, on alveolar bone loss in experimental periodontitis.** The animals were given daily injections of either 0.9% NaCl (control group), or 0.8, 1.6 or 3.2 μmoles/kg (subcutaneous injection) of risedronate (experimental groups) from days 1 to 7, and were killed on day 8. In the control group, histological examination and determination of bone mineral density in the interdental area between 1st and 2nd molars with an image analyzer revealed loss of attachment and bone resorption along with appearance of large number of osteoclasts. However, in the experimental group, the resorption of alveolar bone and the loss of bone mineral content were prevented in a dose dependent manner, especially at doses of 1.6 and 3.2 µmoles/kg. The authors suggested that administration of **risedronate could be effective in preventing bone resorption in periodontitis.**

Kaynak et.al (2003)[124] examined histopathologically the **effect of systemic administration of aminobisphosphonate (alendronate) on alveolar bone resorption following mucoperiosteal flap surgery in rats.** 32 male rats were divided into two groups of 16 rats in each group. The animals were given subcutaneous injections of either saline (control group) or 0.5 mg/kg of alendronate (experimental group). The alendronate or saline was administered subcutaneously 1 week prior to surgery, at the time of surgery, and 1 week after surgery. The parameters determined for histopathological evaluation were as follows: inflammatory cell infiltration (ICI) of adjacent periodontal tissue, degree of fibrosis and collagen bundle formation, number and morphology of osteoclasts of the alveolar bone and interdental septum, resorption lacunae (osteoclast surfaces), and osteoblastic activity (forming surfaces). There were no statistically significant differences between the saline and alendronate groups with regard to inflammatory cell infiltration, number of osteoclasts, and osteoblastic activity. Fibrosis and collagen bundle formation, osteoclast morphologies, and resorption lacunae formation were significantly different between the two groups, in favor of the alendronate group. Based on these findings the authors concluded that the **systemic administration of 0.5 mg/kg alendronate could be effective in preventing alveolar bone loss and in modulating tissue factors.**

Binderman et.al (2000)[122] investigated the effectiveness of different concentrations of alendronate delivery at the surgical site during the time of surgery, and in the cheek mucosa in the opposite side, in reducing alveolar bone loss. 128 wistar rats were divided in two groups: experiment A (60 rats) to explore the effect of different concentrations of alendronate applied at the surgical site at the time of surgery in 2 series of experiments. The second group, experiment B (68 rats), served to explore the effect of different alendronate concentrations delivered at the time of surgery, at a location distant to the surgical site (into the submucosal of the cheek on the contralateral side) in 2 series of experiments. Following elevation of a mucoperiosteal flap, a gelatin sponge soaked with different concentrations of alendronate (0, 1,5,20, or 40 mg/ml; experiment A) was applied to exposed bone on the experimental side. In the second group (experiment B), alendronate (0, 50, 200, or 400 μg) was topically delivered in the cheek mucosa on the left side. The results showed that topical application of 200 μg and 400 μg doses of alendronate at the time of surgery was significantly effective in reducing bone loss. The percentage of sections with mild bone loss increased with an increase in the dose of alendronate, while the percent of sections with severe bone loss decreased with an increase in alendronate dose. They found 200 μg to be effective for topical delivery and 400 μg for distant sites. **The authors concluded that topical delivery of alendronate at the time of surgery reduces bone loss in periodontal procedures.**

Alencar et.al (2002)[123] studied the **effects of administrating disodium chlodronate to rats in an experimental periodontitis model.** Seventy-two male Wistar rats were used for this study. A nylon thread ligature was placed around the left maxillary molars of all rats that were sacrificed after 7 or 11 days. There were 5 groups of 6 animals each for both the prophylactic and curative disodium chlodronate treatments. The disodium chlodronate treatment group received disodium chlodronate (1, 5, or 25 mg/kg), subcutaneously, 1 hour before the surgical procedure and daily until sacrifice at day 7. The curative disodium chlodronate treatment group received disodium chlodronate (1, 5, or 25 mg/kg), subcutaneously 5 days after periodontitis induction and daily until sacrifice at day 11. The non-treated group consisted of 6 animals subjected to experimental periodontal disease which received a saline solution daily and were sacrificed after 7 or 11 days after periodontitis induction. A control group (6 animals) did not receive either disodium chlodronate or saline. The right jaw was used as control. In non-treated group there was significant alveolar bone loss, severe mononuclear cells influx, and increase in osteoclast numbers. Prophylactic disodium chlodronate treatment groups showed decrease alveolar bone loss 25.8 %, 61.6%, and 75.5% as compared to non-treated group for the 1, 5, and 25 mg/kg disodium chlodronate doses, respectively. Curative disodium chlodronate treatment groups showed decrease alveolar bone loss 20%, 62% and 69% as compared to non-treated for the 1, 5, and 25 mg/kg disodium chlodronate doses, respectively. The authors concluded that **disodium chlodronate has both bone sparing and anti-inflammatory activity when administered as a pretreatment or in an ongoing process.**

Ouchi (1998)[121] examined the **efficacy of YM 175 (disodium cycloheptylaminomethylenediphosphonate monohydrate) in reducing alveolar bone loss caused by experimental periodontitis** in beagle dogs. 36 dogs received brushing 3 times a week for 3 months. These were then divided into 6 groups. Periodontitis was induced in the 30 dogs of group 2-6 by ligating the mandibular third and fourth premolars. The animals in group 1 and 2 were given a vehicle, group 3 received flurbiprofen 0.02 mg/kg. Group 4-6 received YM 175 at a dose of 0.01, 0.1 or 1.0 mg/kg orally once a day for 5 days/week. In placebo treated animals (group 2) the ligation caused a significant decrease in alveolar bone height by 0.57 and 1.91 mm at 2 and 25 weeks respectively. YM 175 (1.0 mg/kg) prevented the decrease in bone height by 47 and 31% at 2 and 15 weeks. YM 175 (1.0 mg/kg) and flurbiprofen tended to increase the bone volume. The authors concluded that **YM 175 could prevents alveolar bone loss** by reducing the alveolar bone turnover in dogs with periodontitis.

Lane et.al (2005)[128] carried out a study to determine the **effect of 1 year bisphosphonate therapy in conjunction with conventional non-surgical treatment in patients with moderate to severe chronic periodontitis.** Patients were randomized to the following treatment groups: bisphosphonate (alendronate at 10 mg/day) or risedronate (5mg/day) plus calcium citrate and vitamin D3 or placebo plus calcium citrate and vitamin D3 for 1 year. 70 were randomized, 43 to the bisphosphonate group and 27 to the placebo group. All patients received non-surgical periodontal treatment (scaling, root planing) and periodontal maintenance therapy every 3 months. Clinical assessments at baseline and 6 and 12 months included clinical attachment level (CAL), probing depth (PD), and bleeding on probing (BOP). Periodontal bone mass was assessed by dental radiographs at baseline and 12 months using fractal analysis and digital subtraction radiography (DSR). Bisphosphonate therapy significantly improved CAL, PD, and BOP relative to the placebo group during the 6- to 12-month period. There was no difference in the change in periodontal bone mass between the bisphosphonate and placebo groups as measured by fractal analysis and DSR. The authors concluded that **bisphosphonate treatment may be an appropriate adjunctive treatment to preserve periodontal bone mass** and can lead to improved clinical outcome of non-surgical periodontal therapy.

Rocha et.al (2004)[126] investigated the effect of oral alendronate treatment on radiological and clinical measurements of periodontal disease in postmenopausal women without hormone replacement therapy. 40 postmenopausal women, 55 to 65 years old with established periodontal disease were enrolled in this controlled, double-masked, prospective study. They were randomized to receive alendronate (10 mg/day) or placebo for the 6 months study period. Periodontal mechanical treatment was carried out in both groups. At baseline and after treatment, clinical evaluation, hormone blood levels, distance from the crestal alveolar bone to the cemento-enamel junction

(CEJ), calcaneus bone mineral density (BMD), hormone levels, serum N-telopeptide, and bone-specific alkaline phosphatase were assessed. Greater improvement in probing depth (-0.8 ± 0.3 mm versus -0.4 ± 0.4 mm, and gingival bleeding (-0.3% ± 0.13% versus -0.2% ±0.06%) was found in the alendronate treated group. Calcaneus Crestal alveolar bone increased in the alendronate treated group (68 ± 47 mm^3 versus -26 ± 81 mm^3). Crestal alveolar bone-CEJ distance diminished in the alendronate group (-0.4 ±0.40 mm versus 0.60 ± 0.53 mm). Marginal reduction in both serum N-telopeptide and bone-specific alkaline phosphatase levels was found in the alendronate group (-9.4 ± 6.6 nmol versus -4.3 ± 4.7 nmol bone collagen equivalents and -7.7 +/- 8.4 versus -1.5 +/- 5.0 U/l, respectively). Hormone levels were unchanged after treatment. The authors concluded that **alendronate may be useful in treating periodontal disease in postmenopausal women.**

Takaishi et.al (2003)[125] used intermittent cyclical **etidronate** (etidronate administered orally at a dose of 200 mg/day for 2 weeks, at intervals of 10-12 weeks or 6 months) for 4-5 years in addition to ordinary dental therapy in four women with periodontitis. Alveolar bone density was measured using a new method comparing the percentage increase in density. Mean alveolar bone density was increased significantly during intermittent cyclical etidronate treatment. Significant reductions were observed in the mobility of the teeth and the depth of periodontal pockets. There were significant correlations between alveolar bone density and both mobility of the teeth and the depth of the periodontal pockets. It was reported that **increase in alveolar bone density** was associated with the clinical benefits of etidronate in the treatment of periodontitis.

Gabriela Giro et al (2007)[130] conducted a study which investigated the influence of estrogen deficiency and its treatment with estrogen and **alendronate on the removal torque of osseointegrated titanium implants.** 48 female Wistar rats received a titanium implant in the tibia metaphysis. After

60 days, which was needed for implant osseointegration, the animals were randomly divided into five groups: control (CTLE; N = 10), sham surgery (SHAM; N = 12), ovariectomy (OVX; N = 12), ovariectomy followed by hormone replacement (EST; N = 12), and ovariectomy followed by treatment with alendronate (ALE; N = 12). The CTLE group was sacrificed to confirm osseointegration, whereas the remaining groups were submitted to sham surgery or ovariectomy according to their designations. After 90 days, these animals were also sacrificed. Densitometry of femur and lumbar vertebrae was performed by dual-energy x-ray absorptiometry (DEXA) to confirm systemic impairment of the animals. All implants were subjected to removal torque. Results of densitometric analysis confirmed a systemic impairment of the animals, disclosing lower values of bone mineral density for OVX. Analysis of the removal torque of the implants showed statistically lower values for the OVX group in relation to the other groups. However, the group treated with alendronate (ALE group) presented significantly higher torque values compared to the others. According to this study, **estrogen deficiency was observed to have a negative influence on the removal torque of osseointegrated implants, whereas treatment with alendronate increased the torque needed to remove the implants.**

Juan A. Goya et al (2006)[129] **studied the** effect of topical **administration of monosodium olpadronate (OPD) on experimental periodontitis (EP) in rats. 20 wistar rats were used in this experiment.** The animals were assigned to one of two groups: group I: EP; and group II: EP plus topical administration of OPD (EP + OPD). The contralateral side in both groups served as untreated controls (CI and CII), respectively. Mesio-distally oriented sections of each lower first molar were obtained for histomorphometric evaluation. The treated group (EP + OPD) exhibited marked inhibition of bone loss; interradicular bone volume was significantly greater than that observed in the EP group. Osteoclasts in the OPD treated group were detached from the bone surface, were round in shape, and exhibited a loss of polarity and lack of ruffled borders. The authors concluded that **monosodium olpadronate (OPD) was found to inhibit bone loss and to cause marked morphologic changes in osteoclasts.** The drug effectively prevented bone loss caused by periodontitis.

Several animal studies have examined the effects of local or systemic bisphosphonate delivery on alveolar bone resorption by using the experimental periodontitis model with the observation period in different studies ranged between 7 days to 25 weeks. They have reported significant reduction in bone density changes by using alendronate, however they did not find changes in clinical parameters. This may be attributed to the fact that high-dose release of alendronate from hydroxyapatite in inflamed periodontal pockets upregulated the inflammatory host response by stimulating the secretion of cytokines such as IL-1 and IL-6 (Schweitzer et al. 1995)[127]. However almost the entire study models reported significantly reduced bone loss associated with experimental periodontitis compared with control animals. It was also reported that systemic administration of incadronate had significantly reduced inflammatory cell infiltrations.

Yaff e et al. (1995)[118] reported that when bisphosphonate was applied locally directly onto the exposed alveolar bone during surgery had no noticeable effect on reducing bone resorption, whereas Yaffe et.al (1997)[120] in another study reported marked reduction of bone resorption, maintaining the height of the alveolar crest on topical application of bisphosphonate. The reason for the difference in the results of two studies was probably due to the difference in the concentrations of the drug used and the time period for which the drug was locally applied.

In fact **bisphosphonate therapy has been showed to improve significantly CAL, PD, and BOP in humans during the 6- to 12-month period.** However, in animal studies no significant difference was observed in these clinical parameters. Bisphosphonate therapy also found to improve periodontal bone mass, increase the alveolar bone height, reduce crestal alveolar bone to CEJ distance both in humans and animals. **Palmo L et al (2007)[131]** in a review of bisphosphonate therapy stated that bisphosphonate drugs used for systemic bone loss affect the maxilla and mandible. Alveolar bone loss in periodontitis and skeletal bone loss share common mechanisms. **As bisphosphonate therapy is used for treating various systemic bone diseases it can also be used for treatment of periodontal diseases.** In fact, periodontal therapy using bisphosphonates to modulate host response to bacterial insult may develop into a potential strategy in populations in which periodontal therapy is not convenient. Developing bisphosphonates to slow the progression of periodontal disease depends on identifying an effective dosage regimen and delivery system that would reach the target site in the periodontium, while limiting unwanted side effects. Therefore, the use of bisphosphonate to prevent and/or treat periodontitis must be considered very carefully at this time.

Based on these pre-clinical animal studies and on preliminary human clinical studies, the osteoprotegerin (RANK), RANKL axis is a new target for the treatment of destructive periodontal disease. Further studies are necessary to determine the most efficacious therapeutic approach on this molecular interaction.

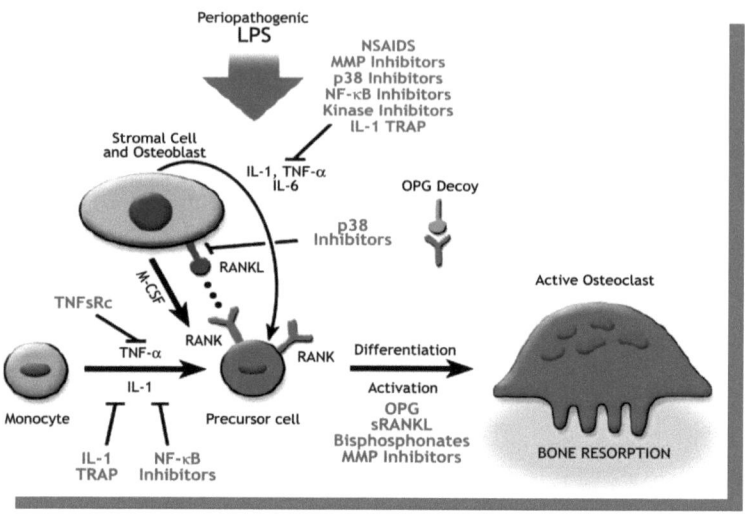

Fig.8. Potential therapeutic strategies to treat bone resorption.

The adjunctive use of HMT with mechanical periodontal therapy has been reported involving non-surgical and surgical approaches. Clinical trials have shown that inhibition of arachidonic acid metabolites with NSAIDs reduces gingival inflammation and periodontal disease progression. However, recently reported serious adverse effects of some COX-2 inhibitors preclude their use as an adjunct to mechanical periodontal therapy. Evidences show that the adjunctive use of SDD to mechanical periodontal therapy down regulates collagenolytic activity and thereby improves the clinical responses above and beyond the result of what is attainable by mechanical intervention. Although there are controversial findings reported on the use of systemic bisphosphonates to prevent periodontal disease progression in human studies, bisphosphonate therapy have been shown to increase osteoblast differentiation, inhibit osteoclast recruitment and activity, and down-regulate activity levels of several MMPs.

Apart from these extensively studied groups of drug newer therapeutic approaches have also been tried. Most of these approaches are still in their infancy and limited to animal experimental studies. The blockade of cytokine receptors (IL-1Ra, TNF-αR1, TNF-αR2) and soluble cytokines (rhIL-11) have demonstrated to reduce periodontal attachment loss and alveolar bone loss by blocking the activity of pro-inflammatory cytokines in animal experimental periodontitis. Similarly, the use of a selective iNOS inhibition mercaptoalkylguanidines has been demonstrated to reduce periodontal attachment and bone loss in animal experimental periodontitis. Also, the use of pharmacological inhibitors of NO and PARP synthase showed promising results. Based on pre-clinical animal studies and on preliminary human clinical studies, the osteoprotegerin/RANK/ RANKL axis is a new target for the treatment of destructive periodontal disease. Osteoprotegerin acts as a decoy receptor, expressed by osteoblastic cells, which binds to RANKL and inhibits osteoclast development. However, further studies are necessary to determine the applicability of these agents as therapeutic drugs.

The use of host modulation therapy in conjunction with anti-biofilm treatments may prove to be advantageous. However this concept need to be validated in controlled clinical trials. As methods that modulate the host response become available, they may be useful as adjunctive therapies for a variety of clinical situations.

SUMMARY & CONCLUSIONS

Bacterial biofilm have been shown to be the primary etiological factor in the initiation of gingival inflammation and subsequent destruction of periodontal tissues. At the same time there is strong evidence that destructive processes occurring as part of the host inflammatory response are responsible for the majority of the hard and soft tissue breakdown leading to the clinical signs of periodontitis. The precise nature of the host inflammatory response is still an area of intense research, but it is clear that host-derived pro-inflammatory mediators and cytokines, together with proteolytic enzymes such as matrix metalloproteinases (MMPs), play a significant role for causing changes in connective tissue and bone metabolism that lead to the breakdown of periodontal ligament (PDL) and alveolar bone resorption. Therefore, the successful long-term management of this disease may require a treatment strategy by integrate therapies that will address both causative components.

To date, non-surgical periodontal treatment has primarily focused on targeting the bacterial burden by mechanical disruption of the subgingival biofilm by SRP or by locally delivered topical antimicrobial agents with SRP to further reduce the bacterial burden. It is clear that standard therapy, such as the removal of supragingival and subgingival plaque and calculus deposits by scaling and root planing has been found to be effective for the majority of the patients associated with periodontitis. However, there is strong evidence that in some patients destructive processes occurring as part of the host inflammatory response are responsible for the periodontal tissue breakdown leading to the clinical signs of periodontitis. Therefore, adjunctive therapeutic agents which modify the destructive nature of the host response to periodontopathogens are potentially valuable to the clinical treatment of periodontitis.

Studies ranging from preclinical animal models to human clinical trials support the basic hypothesis that the inhibition of local arachidonic acid metabolites with nonsteroidal anti-inflammatory drugs (NSAIDs) prevents periodontal disease progression. However, recently reported serious adverse effects of some COX-2 inhibitors preclude their use as an adjunct to mechanical periodontal therapy. Tetracyclines and doxycycline in particular are known to inhibit MMP activities either by direct or indirect non-antimicrobial mechanism, thus preventing connective tissue breakdown and bone resorption. Evidence shows that non-surgical periodontal therapy with an adjunctive use of 20 mg SDD twice daily for 9 months was shown to down-regulate collagenolytic activity and thereby improvement in clinical response. Recently bisphosphonate therapy has been tried to prevent periodontal disease progression due to its ability to inhibit osteoclast recruitment and down-regulate levels of several MMPs. However, controversial data on the effects of systemic bisphosphonate administration to prevent periodontal disease progression have been reported both in animal experiments and human studies.

In addition to these extensively studied groups of drugs newer therapeutic approaches have also been tried. Most of these approaches are still in the infancy and limited to animal experimental studies only. Investigations on use of soluble protein delivery of antagonists to interleukin-1 and tumor necrosis factor in a primate model of periodontitis have shown promising results by blocking progression of inflammatory cell infiltrate towards the alveolar crest, thereby preventing periodontal attachment loss. Similarly, the use of, a pharmacological inhibitor of NO and PARP synthatase showed promising result in reducing periodontal attachment loss. Recently, it has been suggested that diagnosis of active bone loss by measuring the ratio of receptor activator of nuclear factor-kappa B ligand (RANKL)/osteoprotegerin (OPG) may prove to be a novel diagnostic parameter.[174] However, further studies are necessary to determine the applicability of these agents as therapeutic drugs. It is conceived that a new potential agents to modulate host response may be developed in future.

REFERENCES

1. Kenneth Korman .Mapping the pathogenesis of periodontitis-A new look.J Periodontol 2008; 79:1560-1568.

2. Dana Graves et al. Cytokines that promote periodontal tissue destruction.J Periodontol 2008; 79:1585-1591.

3. Thomas Van Dyke. Management of inflammation in periodontal diseases. J.Periodontol 2008;79:1601-1608.

4. Maria Emanuel Ryan. Connective Tissues of periodontium; research & clinical ramifications. Perio 2000, Vol 24;2000:227-234.

5. Ian L.C. Chapple, John.B. Matthews.Role of reactive oxygen & antioxidant species in periodontal tissue destruction. Perio 2000, Vol 43; 2007:163-230.

6. Kantarci A, Van Dyke TE. Lipoxins in chronic inflammation. Crit Rev Oral Biol Med 2003; 14 (1):4-12.

7. Trepicchio WL, Bozza M, Pedneult G, Dorner AJ. Recombinant human IL-11 attenuates the inflammatory response through down regulation of pro-inflammatory cytokines release and nitric oxide production. Cited by Keith L. Kirkwood, Joni A. Cirelli, Jill E. Rogers and Williams V. Giannobile. Novel Host Response Therapeutic Approaches to treat periodontal diseases in Periodontol 2000. Vol 43; 2007; 294-315.

8. William V.Giannobile. Host-Response Therapeutics for Periodontal Diseases. J.Periodontol 2008; 79:1592-1600.

9. Page RC. & Kornman KS. The pathogenesis of human periodontitis: an introduction. Periodontol 2000; 1997: 14, 9–11.

10. Graves DT. & Cochran, D. L. The contribution of interleukin-1 and tumor necrosis factor to periodontal tissue destruction. J Periodontol 2003; 74: 391–401.

11. Reynolds JJ. & Meickle, M. C. Mechanisms of connective tissue matrix destruction in periodontitis. Periodontol 2000 1997; 14:144–157.

12. Offenbacher S. Periodontal Diseases: Pathogenesis. Ann Periodontol 1996; 1: 821 – 878.

13. Offenbacher S, Peter A. Heasman, and John G. Collins Modulation of Host PGE2 Secretion as a Determinant of Periodontal Disease Expression. J Periodontol 1993; 64:432-444.

14. Nathan C. Perspective series: Nitric oxide and nitric oxide synthase. Inducible nitric oxide synthase: What difference does it make? Cited by Berdeli A, Gurkan A, Emingil G, Atilla G, and Kose T. Endothelial Nitric Oxide Synthase Glu298Asp Gene Polymorphism in Periodontal Diseases in J Periodontol 2006; 77: 1348-1354.

15. Lyons CR. The role of nitric oxide in inflammation. Cited by Gullu C, Ozmeric N, Tokman B, Elgun S, Balos K. Effectiveness Of Scaling And Root Planing Versus modified Widman flap on Nitric Oxide Synthase

And Arginase Activity In Patients With Chronic Periodontitis in J Periodont Res 2005; 40: 168-175.

16. McCauley LK and Nohutcu RM. Mediators of Periodontal Osseous Destruction and Remodeling: Principles and Implications for Diagnosis and Therapy. J Periodontol 2002; 73: 1377-1391.

17. Gierse JK., Hauser SD., Creely DP., Rangwala SH., Isakson P. C. & Seibert K. Expression and selective inhibition of the constitutive and inducible forms of human cyclo-oxygenase. Cited by Salvi GE, Lang NP. Host response modulation in the management of periodontal diseases in J Clin Peridontol 2005; 32 (Suppl. 6): 108–129.

18. Morton, R. S. & Dongari-Bagtzoglou, A.I. Cyclooxygenase-2 is upregulated in inflamed gingival tissues. J Periodontol 2001; 72, 461–469.

19. Miyauchi, M., Hiraoka, M., Oka, H., Sato, S., Kudo, Y., Ogawa, I., Noguchi, K., Ishikawa, I. & Takata, T. Immuno-localization of COX-1 and COX-2 in the rat molar periodontal tissue after topical application of lipopolysaccharide. Cited by Salvi GE, Lang NP. Host response modulation in the management of periodontal diseases in J Clin Peridontol 2005; 32 (Suppl. 6): 108–129.

20. de Leval X., Hanson, J., David, J. L., Masereel, B., Pirotte, B. & Dogne, J. M. New developments on thromboxane and prostacyclin modulators part II: prostacyclin modulators. Cited by Salvi GE, Lang NP. Host response modulation in the management of periodontal diseases in J Clin Peridontol 2005; 32 (Suppl. 6): 108–129.

21. Neuman SD. & Raisz LG. Effects of the prostaglandin products 6-keto prostaglandin E1 and 6-keto prostaglandin F1a on bone resorption in vitro. Cited by Salvi GE, Lang NP. Host response modulation in the management of periodontal diseases in J Clin Peridontol 2005; 32 (Suppl. 6): 108–129.

22. Birkedal-Hansen H. Role of cytokines and inflammatory mediators in tissue destruction. J Periodont Res 1993;28:500–510.

23. Offenbacher S, Peter A. Heasman, and John G. Collins Modulation of Host PGE2 Secretion as a Determinant of Periodontal Disease Expression. J Periodontol 1993; 64:432-444.

24. Bandeira-Melo C, Bozza PT, Weller PF. The cellular biology of eosinophil eicosanoid formation and function. Cited by Alpdogan Kantarci, Thomas E. Van Dyke. Lipoxins in Chronic Inflammation in Crit Rev Oral Biol Med 2003; 14(1):4-12.

25. Lehr HA, Olofsson AM, Carew TE, Vajkoczy P, von Andrian UH, Hubner C, *et al.* (1994). P-selectin mediates the interaction of circulating leukocytes with platelets and microvascular endothelium in response to oxidized lipoprotein *in vivo*. Cited by Alpdogan Kantarci, Thomas E. Van Dyke. Lipoxins in Chronic Inflammation in Crit Rev Oral Biol Med 2003; 14(1):4-12.

26. Borgeat P., and Samuelsson B.: Transformation of arachidonic acid by rabbit polymorphonuclear leukocytes. Formation of a novel dihydroxyeicosatetraenoic acid. Cited by Offenbacher S, Steven S. Scott, Bonnie M. Odle, Carolyn Wilson-Burrows and Thomas E, Van Dyke.

Depressed Leukotriene B4 Chemotactic Response of Neutrophils from Localized Juvenile Periodontitis Patients. J Periodontol 1987; 602 – 606.

27. Goetzl EJ., Brindley LL, Goldman DW.: Enhancement of human neutrophil adherence by synthetic leukotriene constituents of the slow-reacting substance of anaphylaxis. Cited by Offenbacher S, Steven S. Scott, Bonnie M. Odle, Carolyn Wilson-Burrows and Thomas E, Van Dyke. Depressed Leukotriene B4 Chemotactic Response of Neutrophils from Localized Juvenile Periodontitis Patients in J Periodontol 1987; 602 – 606.

28. Cheng X, Kinosaki M, Murali R, Greene MI, The TNF receptor super-family: Role in immune inflammation and bone formation. Cited by Keith L. Kirkwood, Joni A. Cirelli, Jill E. Rogers and Williams V. Giannobile. Novel Host Response Therapeutic Approaches to treat periodontal diseases in Periodontol 2000. Vol 43; 2007; 294-315.

29. Meghji S., Sandy JR., Scutt AM., Harvey W. & Harris M. Stimulation of bone resorption by lipoxygenase metabolites of arachidonic acid. Cited by Meghji S, Brian Henderson, Sean Nair, and Michael Wilson. Inhibition of Bone DNA and Collagen Production by Surface-Associated Material from Bacteria Implicated in the Pathology of Periodontal Disease in J Periodontol 1992; 63:736-742.

30. Gallwitz WE., Mundy GR., Lee CH., Qiao M., Roodman GD., Raftery M., Gaskell SJ. & Bonewald L. F. 5- lipoxygenase metabolites of arachidonic acid stimulate isolated osteclasts to resorb calcified matrices. Cited by Drisko C.H. Non-Surgical Pocket Therapy: Pharmacotherapeutics in Annals Periodontol 1996; 1: 491 – 566.

31. Diamond P, McGinty A, Sugrue D, Brady HR, Godson C. Regulation of leukocyte trafficking by lipoxins. Cited by Alpdogan Kantarci, Thomas E. Van Dyke. Lipoxins in Chronic Inflammation in Crit Rev Oral Biol Med 2003; 14(1):4-12.

32. Edenius C, Stenke L, Lindgren A. On the mechanism of transcellular lipoxin formation in human platelets and granulocytes. Cited by Alpdogan Kantarci, Thomas E. Van Dyke. Lipoxins in Chronic Inflammation in Crit Rev Oral Biol Med 2003; 14(1):4-12.

33. Serhan CN. Lipoxin biosynthesis and its impact in inflammatory and vascular events. Cited by Alpdogan Kantarci, Thomas E. Van Dyke. Lipoxins in Chronic Inflammation in Crit Rev Oral Biol Med 2003; 14(1):4-12.

34. Levy BD, Clish CB, Schmidt B, Gronert K, Serhan CN. Lipid mediator class switching during acute inflammation: signals in resolution. Cited by Alpdogan Kantarci, Thomas E. Van Dyke. Lipoxins in Chronic Inflammation in Crit Rev Oral Biol Med 2003; 14(1):4-12.

35. Serhan CN, Hamberg M, Samuelsson B. Lipoxins: novel series of biologically active compounds formed from arachidonic acid in human leukocytes. Cited by Alpdogan Kantarci, Thomas E. Van Dyke. Lipoxins in Chronic Inflammation in Crit Rev Oral Biol Med 2003; 14(1):4-12.

36. Hutchinson AW. Arachidonate 15-lipoxygenase: characteristics and potential biological significance. Cited by Alpdogan Kantarci, Thomas E. Van Dyke. Lipoxins in Chronic Inflammation in Crit Rev Oral Biol Med 2003; 14(1):4-12.

37. Serhan CN, Ashish Jain, Sylvie Marleau, Clary Clish, Alpdogan Kantarci, Balsam Behbehani, Sean P. Colgan, Gregory L. Stahl, Aksam Merched, Nicos A. Petasis, Lawrence Chan and Thomas E. Van Dyke. Reduced Inflammation and Tissue Damage in Transgenic Rabbits Overexpressing 15-Lipoxygenase and Endogenous Anti-inflammatory Lipid Mediators. Cited by Salvi GE, Lang NP. Host response modulation in the management of periodontal diseases in J Clin Peridontol 2005; 32 (Suppl. 6): 108–129.

38. Fiore S, Serhan CN (1990). Formation of lipoxins and leukotrienes during receptor mediated interactions of human platelets andrecombinant human granulocyte/macrophage colony-stimulating factor-primed neutrophils. Cited by Alpdogan Kantarci, Thomas E. Van Dyke. Lipoxins in Chronic Inflammation in Crit Rev Oral Biol Med 2003; 14(1):4-12.

39. Claria J, Serhan CN. Aspirin triggers previously undescribed bioactive eicosanoids by human endothelial cell-leukocyte interactions. Cited by Alpdogan Kantarci, Thomas E. Van Dyke. Lipoxins in Chronic Inflammation in Crit Rev Oral Biol Med 2003; 14(1):4-12.

40. Herschman HR (1996). Prostaglandin synthase 2. Cited by Alpdogan Kantarci, Thomas E. Van Dyke. Lipoxins in Chronic Inflammation in Crit Rev Oral Biol Med 2003; 14(1):4-12.

41. Hachicha M, Pouliot M, Petasis NA, Serhan CN (1999). Lipoxin A4 and aspirin-triggered 15-epi-LXA4 inhibit tumor necrosis factor- initiated neutrophil responses and trafficking: regulators of a cytokine-chemokine axis. Cited by Alpdogan Kantarci, Thomas E. Van Dyke. Lipoxins in Chronic Inflammation in Crit Rev Oral Biol Med 2003; 14(1):4-12.

42. Pouliot M, Clish CB, Petasis NA, Van Dyke TE, Serhan CN. Lipoxin A4 analogues inhibit leukocyte recruitment to *Porphyromonas gingivalis*: a role for cyclooxygenase-2 and lipoxins in periodontal disease. Cited by Alpdogan Kantarci, Thomas E. Van Dyke. Lipoxins in Chronic Inflammation in Crit Rev Oral Biol Med 2003; 14(1):4-12.

43. Birkedal-Hansen. Role of Matrix Metalloproteinases in Human Periodontal Diseases. J Periodontol 1993; 64:474-484.

44. Reynolds JJ. & Meickle, M. C. Mechanisms of connective tissue matrix destruction in periodontitis. Periodontol 2000 1997; 14:144–157.

45. Birkedal-Hansen, H., Moore, W. G., Bodden, M. K., Windsor, L. J., Birkedal-Hansen, B., DeCarlo, A. & Engler, J. A. Matrix metalloproteinases: a review. Cited by Salvi GE, Lang NP. Host response modulation in the management of periodontal diseases in J Clin Peridontol 2005; 32 (Suppl. 6): 108–129.

46. Yaffe A., Fine N., Alt I. & Binderman I. The effect of bisphosphonate on alveolar bone resorption following mucoperiosteal flap surgery in the mandible of rats. J Periodontol 1995; 66: 999–1003.

47. MacNaul K. L., Chartrain, N., Lark, M., Tocci, M. J. & Hutchinson, N. I. Discoordinate expression of stromelysin, collagenase, and tissue inhibitor of metalloproteinases-1 in rheumatoid human synovial fibroblasts. Cited by Preshaw PM, Hefti AF, Jepsen S, Etienne D, Walker C, Bradshaw MH Subantimicrobial dose doxycycline as adjunctive treatment for periodontitis in J Clin Periodontol 2004; 31: 697–707.

48. Caton JG, Ciancio, S. G., Blieden, T. M.,Bradshaw, M., Crout, R. J., Hefti, A. F., Massaro, J. M., Polson, A. M., Thomas, J. & Walker, C. Treatment with subantimicrobial dose doxycycline improves the efficacy of scaling and root planing in patients with adult periodontitis. J Periodontol 2000; 71:521–532.

49. Sorsa T., Uitto VJ., Suomalainen K., Vauhkonen M. & Lindy S. Comparison of interstitial collagenases from human gingiva, sulcular fluid and polymorphonuclear leukocytes. J Periodont Res 1988; 23: 386–393.

50. Golub LM., Ryan, M. E. & Williams, R. C. Modulation of the host response in the treatment of periodontitis. Cited by Preshaw PM, Hefti AF, Jepsen S, Etienne D, Walker C, Bradshaw MH Subantimicrobial dose doxycycline as adjunctive treatment for periodontitis in J Clin Periodontol 2004; 31: 697–707.

51. Mariotti A. The extracellular matrix of the periodontium: dynamic and interactive tissues. Periodontol 2000 1993 Oct; 3:39-63. Review.

52. Uitto VJ., Airola, K., Vaalamo, M., Johansson, N., Putnins, E. E., Firth, J. D., Salonen, J., Lopez-Otin, C., Saarialho-Kere, U. & Kahari, V. M (1998). Collagenase-3 (matrix metalloproteinase-13) expression is induced in oral mucosal epithelium during chronic inflammation. Cited by Preshaw PM, Hefti AF, Jepsen S, Etienne D, Walker C, Bradshaw MH Subantimicrobial dose doxycycline as adjunctive treatment for periodontitis in J Clin Periodontol 2004; 31: 697–707.

53. Ejeil AL., Igondjo-Tchen, S., Ghomrasseni, S., Pellat, B., Godeau, G. & Gogly, B. Expression of matrix metalloproteinases (MMPs) and tissue

inhibitors of metalloproteinases (TIMPs) in healthy and diseased human gingiva. J Periodontol 2003; 74: 188–195.

54. Kinane DF., Darby, I. B., Said, S., Luoto, H., Sorsa, T., Tikanoja, S. & Mantyla, P. Changes in gingival crevicular fluid matrix metalloproteinase-8 levels during periodontal treatment and maintenance. J Periodont Res. 2003; 38:400–404.

55. Wucherpfennig AL, Li YP, Stetler-Stevenson WG, Rosenberg AE, Stashenko P. Expression of 92 kD type IV collagenase/gelatinase B in human osteoclasts. J Bone Miner Res. 1994 Apr;9(4):549-56.

56. Gamonal J, Acevedo A, Bascones A, Jorge O, Silva A. Levels of interleukin-1 beta, -8, and -10 and RANTES in gingival crevicular fluid and cell populations in adult periodontitis patients and the effect of periodontal treatment. J Periodontol 2000: 71; 1535-1545.

57. Hirano T, Akira S, Taga T, Kishimoto T Biological and clinical aspects of interleukin-6. Cited by Dimitris N. Tatakis Interleukin-1 and Bone Metabolism: A Review in J Periodontol 1993; 64:416-431.

58. Dinarello CA. Therapeutic strategies to reduce IL-1 activity in treating local and systemic inflammation. Cited by Salvi GE, Lang NP. Host response modulation in the management of periodontal diseases in J Clin Peridontol 2005; 32 (Suppl. 6): 108–129.

59. Okada S, Inoue H, Yamauchi K, et.al. Potential role of interleukin-1 allergen induced late asthamatic reactions in guinea pigs: Suppressive effect of interleukin-1 receptor antagonist on late asthamatic reaction.

Cited by Graves, D. T. & Cochran, D. L. The contribution of interleukin-1 and tumor necrosis factor to periodontal tissue destruction in J Periodontol 2003; 74: 391–401.

60. Dudley D. Pre-term labor: An intr-uterine inflammatory response syndrome? Cited by Graves, D. T. & Cochran, D. L. The contribution of interleukin-1 and tumor necrosis factor to periodontal tissue destruction in J Periodontol 2003; 74: 391–401.

61. Franceschi RT. The development control of osteoblast - specific gene expression: role of specific transcription factor and the extracellular matrix environment. Cited by McCauley LK and Nohutcu RM. Mediators of Periodontal Osseous Destruction and Remodeling: Principles and Implications for Diagnosis and Therapy in J Periodontol 2002; 73: 1377-1391.

62. Dimitris N. Tatakis Interleukin-1 and Bone Metabolism: A Review. J Periodontol 1993; 64:416-431.

63. Hirano T, Akira S, Taga T, Kishimoto T Biological and clinical aspects of interleukin-6. Cited by Dimitris N. Tatakis Interleukin-1 and Bone Metabolism: A Review in J Periodontol 1993; 64:416-431.

64. Bartold PM, Haynes DR. Interleukin-6 production by human gingival fibroblasts. J Periodont Res 1991; 26:339–345. Gallwitz WE., Mundy GR., Lee CH., Qiao M., Roodman GD., Raftery M., Gaskell SJ. & Bonewald L. F. 5- lipoxygenase metabolites of arachidonic acid stimulate isolated osteclasts to resorb calcified matrices. Cited by Drisko C.H. Non-Surgical

Pocket Therapy: Pharmacotherapeutics in Annals Periodontol 1996; 1: 491 – 566.

65. De Waal Malefyt R., Abrams, J., Bennett, B., Figdor, C. & de Vries, J. Interleukin-10 (IL-10) inhibits cytokine synthesis by human monocytes: an autoregulatory role of IL-10 produced by monocytes. Cited by Salvi GE, Lang NP. Host response modulation in the management of periodontal diseases in J Clin Peridontol 2005; 32 (Suppl. 6): 108–129.

66. Trepicchio WL, Bozza M, Pedneult G, Dorner AJ. Recombinant human IL-11 attenuates the inflammatory response through down regulation of pro-inflammatory cytokines release and nitric oxide production. Cited by Keith L. Kirkwood, Joni A. Cirelli, Jill E. Rogers and Williams V. Giannobile. Novel Host Response Therapeutic Approaches to treat periodontal diseases in Periodontol 2000. Vol 43; 2007; 294-315.

67. Castro L, Rodrigouez M. Aconitase is resdily inactivated by by peroxynitrite, but only by its precursor,nitric oxide J Biol Chem 1994:269: 29409-29415.

68. Murrell GA, Jang D, Williams RJ. Nitric oxide activates metalloprotease enzymes in articular cartilage. Cited by Daghigh, F., Borghaei, R. C., Thornton, R. D. & Bee, J. H. Human gingival fibroblasts produce nitric oxide in response to proinflammatory cytokines in J Periodontol 2002; 73, 392–400.

69. Brennan PA., Thomas G. J. & Langdon J. D. The role of nitric oxide in oral diseases. Cited by Gullu C, Ozmeric N, Tokman B, Elgun S, Balos K. Effectiveness Of Scaling And Root Planing Versus modified Widman flap

on Nitric Oxide Synthase And Arginase Activity In Patients With Chronic Periodontitis in J Periodont Res 2005; 40: 168-175.

70. Matejka M, Partyka L, Ulm C, Solar P, Sinzinger H. Nitric oxide synthase is increased in periodontal disease. J Periodont Res 1998; 33:517-518.

71. Manolagas SC. Birth and death of bone cells: basic regulatory mechanisms and implications for the pathogenesis and treatment of osteoporosis. Cited by McCauley LK and Nohutcu RM. Mediators of Periodontal Osseous Destruction and Remodeling: Principles and Implications for Diagnosis and Therapy in J Periodontol 2002; 73: 1377-1391.

72. Gierse JK., Hauser SD., Creely DP., Rangwala SH., Isakson P. C. & Seibert K. Expression and selective inhibition of the constitutive and inducible forms of human cyclo-oxygenase. Cited by Salvi GE, Lang NP. Host response modulation in the management of periodontal diseases in J Clin Peridontol 2005; 32 (Suppl. 6): 108–129.

73. Teng YT, Nguyen H, Gao X, Kong YY, Gorczynski RM, Singh B, Ellen RP, Penninger JM. Functional human T-cell immunity and osteoprotegerin ligand control alveolar bone destruction in periodontal infection. Cited by Keith L. Kirkwood, Joni A. Cirelli, Jill E. Rogers and Williams V. Giannobile. Novel Host Response Therapeutic Approaches to treat periodontal diseases in Periodontol 2000. Vol 43; 2007; 294-315.

74. Fieldman RS, Betty Szento, Howard H. Chauncey, and Paul Goldhaber. Non-steroidal anti-inflammatory drugs in the reduction of human alveolar bone loss. J Clin Periodontol 1983; 10: 131-136.

75. Heasman PA, Seymour RA and Boston PP: The effect of a topical non-steroidal anti-inflammatory drug on the development of experimental gingivitis in man J Clin Periodontol 1989: 16: 353-358.

76. Williams R C., Marjorie K. Jeffcoat, T. Howard Howell, Arturo Rolla, Derek Stubbs, Kok W. Teoh, Michael S. Reddy, and Paul Goldhaber. Altering the progression of Human alveolar Bone Loss with the Non-Steroidal Anti-Inflammatory Drug Flurbiprofen. J Periodontol 1989; 60:485-490.

77. Reddy MS., Palcanis, K. G., Barnett, M. L., Haigh, S., Charles, C. H. & Jeffcoat, M. K. Efficacy of meclofenamate sodium (Meclomen) in the treatment of rapidly progressive periodontitis. J Clin Periodontol 1993; 20:635–640.

78. Heasman, P. A., Offenbacher, S., Collins, J. G., Edwards, G. & Seymour, R. A. Flurbiprofen in the prevention and treatment of experimental gingivitis. J Clin Periodontol 1993b; 20:732–738.

79. Heasman, PA., Seymour, R. A. & Kelly, P. J. The effect of systemically administered flurbiprofen as an adjunct to toothbrushing on the resolution of experimental gingivitis. J Clin Periodontol 1994; 21: 166–170.

80. Jeffcoat, M. K., Reddy, M. S., Haigh, S., Buchanan, W., Doyle, M. J., Meredith, M. P., Nelson, S. L., Goodale, M. B. & Wehmeyer, K. R. A comparison of topical ketorolac, systemic flurbiprofen, and placebo for the inhibition of bone loss in adult periodontitis. J Periodontol 1995; 66:329–338.

81. Preshaw, P. M., Lauffart, B., Brown, P., Zak, E. & Heasman, P. A. Efffects of ketorolac tromethamine mouthrinse (0.1%) on crevicular fluid prostaglandin E2 concentrations in untreated chronic periodontitis. J Periodontol 1998; 69: 777–783.

82. Bichara J., Greenwell, H., Drisko, C., Wittwer, J. W., Vest, T. M., Yancey, J., Goldsmith, J. & Rebitski, G. The effect of postsurgical naproxen and a bioabsorbable membrane on osseous healing in intrabony defects. J Periodontol 1999; 70: 869–877.

83. Pouliot M, Serhan CN. Lipoxin A4 and aspirin-triggered 15-epi-LXA4 inhibit tumor necrosis factor-alpha-initiated neutrophil responses and trafficking: novel regulators of a cytokine-chemokine axis relevant to periodontal diseases. J Periodont Res. 1999 Oct; 34(7): 370-3.

84. Bezerra, M. M., de Lima, V., Alencar, V. B. M. Vieira, I. B., Brito, G. A. C., Ribeiro, R. A. & Rocha, F. A. Selective cyclooxygenase-2 inhibition prevents alveolar bone loss in experimental periodontitis in rats. J Periodontol 2000; 71: 1009–1014.

85. Paquette, D. W., Lawrence, H. P., McCombs, G. B., Wilder, R., Binder, T. A., Troullos, E., Annett, M., Friedman, M., Smith, P. C. & Offenbacher, S. Pharmacodynamic effects of ketoprofen on crevicular fluid prostanoids in adult periodontitis. J Clin Periodontol 2000; 27: 558–566.

86. Holzhausen, M., Rossa, C. Jr., Marcantonio, E. Jr., Nassar, P. O., Spolidorio, D. M. P. & Spolidorio, L. C. Effect of selective cyclooxygenase-2 inhibition on the development of ligature-induced periodontitis in rats. J Periodontol 2002; 73:1030–1036.

87. Vardar, S., Baylas, H. & Huseyinov, A. Effects of selective cyclooxygenase-2 inhibition on gingival tissue levels of prostaglandin E2 and prostaglandin F2a and clinical parameters of chronic periodontitis. J Periodontol 2003; 74: 57–63.

88. Serhan CN, Ashish Jain, Sylvie Marleau, Clary Clish, Alpdogan Kantarci, Balsam Behbehani, Sean P. Colgan, Gregory L. Stahl, Aksam Merched, Nicos A. Petasis, Lawrence Chan and Thomas E. Van Dyke. Reduced Inflammation and Tissue Damage in Transgenic Rabbits Overexpressing 15-Lipoxygenase and Endogenous Anti-inflammatory Lipid Mediators. Cited by Salvi GE, Lang NP. Host response modulation in the management of periodontal diseases in J Clin Peridontol 2005; 32 (Suppl. 6): 108–129.

89. Gurgel de Vasconcelos, B. C., Duarte, P. M., Nociti, F. H. Jr., Sallum, E. A., Casati, M. Z., Sallum, A. W. & de Toledo, S. Impact of an anti-inflammatory therapy and its withdrawal on the progression of experimental periodontitis in rats. J Periodontol 2004; 75:1613–1618.

90. Sekino S., Ramberg, P. & Lindhe, J. The effect of systemic administration of ibuprofen in the experimental gingivitis model. J Clin Periodontol 2005; 32:182–187.

91. Kurtis B, Gulay Tuter, Muhittin Serdar, Selin Pinar, Ilkim Demirel, Utku Toyman. Gingival Crevicular Fluid Prostaglandin E2 and Thiobarbituric Acid Reactive Substance Levels in Smokers and Non-Smokers With Chronic Periodontitis Following Phase I Periodontal Therapy and Adjunctive Use of Flurbiprofen. J Periodontol 2007; 78: 104-111.

92. C. Alec Yen, Petros D. Damoulis. The Effect of a Selective Cyclooxygenase-2 Inhibitor (Celecoxib) on Chronic Periodontitis. J.Periodontol, 2008, Vol. 79, No. 1, Pages 104-113.

93. Thais M. Oliveira,* Vivien T. Sakai. COX-2 Inhibition Decreases VEGF Expression and Alveolar Bone Loss During the Progression of Experimental Periodontitis in Rats. J.Periodontol, 2008, Vol 79, No.6:1062-1069.

94. Golub LM., Sorsa, T., Lee, H. M., Ciancio, S., Sorbi, D., Ramamurthy, N. S., Gruber, B., Salo, T. & Konttinen, Y. T. Doxycycline inhibits neutrophil (PMN)-type matrix metallopreteinases in human adult periodontitis gingiva. J Clin Periodontol 1995; 22: 100–109.

95. Crout RJ., Lee, H. M., Schroeder, K., Crout, H., Ramamurthy, N. S., Wiener, M. & Golub, L. M. The "cyclic" regimen of low dose doxycycline for adult periodontitis: a preliminary study. J Periodontol 1996; 67: 506–514.

96. Veronica W-K Ng and Nabil F. Bissada clinical evaluation of systemic doxycycline and ibuprofen administration as an adjunctive treatment for adult periodontitis. J Periodontol 1998; 69:772-776.

97. Caton JG, Ciancio, S. G., Blieden, T. M.,Bradshaw, M., Crout, R. J., Hefti, A. F., Massaro, J. M., Polson, A. M., Thomas, J. & Walker, C. Treatment with subantimicrobial dose doxycycline improves the efficacy of scaling and root planing in patients with adult periodontitis. J Periodontol 2000; 71:521–532.

98. H.Nakaya, G.Osawa. Effects of bisphosphonates on matrix metalloproteinases enzymes in periodontal ligament cells.J.Periodontol, July 2000, Vol. 71, No. 7, Pages 1158-1166.

99. Golub LM, McNamara, T. F., Ryan, M. E., Kohut, B., Blieden, T., Payonk, G., Sipos, T. & Baron, H. J. Adjunctive treatment, with subantimicrobial doses of doxycycline: effects on gingival fluid collagenase activity and attachment loss in adult periodontitis. J Clin Periodontol 2001; 28,146–156.

100. Ramamurthy NS, Rifkin, B. R., Greenwald, R. A., Xu, J.-W., Liu, Y., Turner, G., Golub, L. M. & Vernillo, A. T. Inhibition of matrix metalloproteinase-mediated periodontal bone loss in rats: a comparison of 6 chemically modified tetracyclines. J Periodontol 2002a; 73:726–734.

101. Novak MJ, Johns, L. P., Miller, R. C. & Bradshaw, M. H. Adjunctive benefits of subantimicrobial dose doxycycline in the management of severe, generalized, chronic periodontitis. J Periodontol 2002; 73:762–769.

102. Emingil G, Atilla, G., Sorsa, T., Luoto, H., Kirilmaz, L. & Baylas, H. The effect of adjunctive low-dose doxycycline therapy on clinical parameters and gingival crevicular fluid matrix metalloproteinase-8 levels in chronic periodontitis. J Periodontol 2004a; 75:106–115.

103. Gapski R, Barr, J. L., Sarment, D. P., Layher, M. G., Socransky, S. S. & Giannoblle, W. V. Effect of systemic matrix metalloproteinase inhibition on periodontal wound repair: a proof of concept trial. J Periodontol 2004; 75:441–452.

104. Gurkan A, Cinarcik S, Huseyinov A. Adjunctive subantimicrobial dose doxycycline: effect on clinical parameters and gingival crevicular fluid transforming growth factor - β1 levels in severe, generalized chronic periodontitis. J Clin Periodontol 2005; 32: 244–253.

105. Preshaw PM, Heasman L, Stacey F, Steen N, McCracken GI, Heasman PA. The effect of quitting smoking on chronic periodontitis. J Clin Periodontol. 2005 Aug; 32(8):869-79.

106. Buduneli N, Buduneli E, Cinar S, Lappin D, Kinane DF. Immunohistochemical evaluation of Ki-67 expression and apoptosis in cyclosporin A-induced gingival overgrowth. J Periodontol 2007; 78(2): 282-9.

107. G.Emingil, Gul Atilla. The Effect of Adjunctive Subantimicrobial Dose Doxycycline Therapy on GCF EMMPRIN Levels in Chronic Periodontitis. J.Periodontol 2008, Vol. 79, No. 3, Pages 469-476.

108. LM.Golub, HM Lee,Subantimicrobial Dose-Doxycycline modulates gingival crevicular fluid biomarkers of periodontitis in post menopausal osteopenic women.J.Periodontol,2008:79:No.8;1409-1418.

109. Assuma R., Oates, T., Cochran, D. L., Amar, S. & Graves, D. T. IL-1 and TNF antagonists inhibit the inflammatory response and bone loss in experimental periodontitis. Cited by Salvi GE, Lang NP. Host response modulation in the management of periodontal diseases in J Clin Peridontol 2005; 32 (Suppl. 6): 108–129.

110. Graves DT., Delima, A. J., Assuma, R., Amar, S., Oates, T. & Cochran, D. L. Interleukin-1 and tumor necrosis factor antagonists inhibit the progression of inflammatory cell infiltration toward alveolar bone in experimental periodontitis. J Periodontol 1998; 69:1419–1425.

111. Lohinai Z., Benedek, P., Feher, E., Gyorfi, A., Rosivall, L., Fazekas, A., Salzman, A. L. & Szabo, C. Protective effects of mercaptoethylguanidine, a selective inhibitor of inducible nitric oxide synthase, in ligatureinduced periodontitis in the rat. Cited by Salvi GE, Lang NP. Host response modulation in the management of periodontal diseases in J Clin Peridontol 2005; 32 (Suppl. 6): 108–129.

112. Martuscelli G, Fiorellini, J. P., Crohin, C. C. & Howell, T. H. The effect of interleukin- 11 on the progression of ligature-induced periodontal disease in the beagle dog. J Periodontol 2000; 71: 573–578.

113. Delima AJ., Oates, T., Assuma, R., Schwarzt, Z., Cochran, D. L., Amar, S. & Graves, D. T. Soluble antagonists to interleukin-1 (IL-1) and tumor necrosis factor (TNF) inhibits loss of tissue attachment in experimental periodontitis. J Clin Periodontol 2001; 28: 233–240.

114. Oates TW, Graves DT, Cochran DL: Clinical, radiographic and biochemical assessment of IL-1/TNF-a antagonist inhibition of bone loss in experimental periodontitis. J Clin Periodontol 2002; 29: 137–143.

115. Lohinai Z., Mabley, J. G., Feher, E., Marton, A., Komjati, K. & Szabo, C. Role of the activation of the nuclear enzyme poly(-ADP-ribose) polymerase in the pathogenesis of periodontitis. J Dent Res 2003; 82: 987–992.

116. Brunsvold MA., Chaves ES., Kornman KS., Aufdemorte TB. & Wood R. Effects of a bisphosphonate on experimental periodontitis in monkeys. J Periodontol 1992; 63: 825–830.

117. Weinreb M., Quartuccio H., Seedor JG., Aufdemorte TB., Brunsvold M., Chaves E., Kornman K. S. & Rodan G. A. Histomorphometrical analysis of the effects of the bisphosphonate alendronate on bone loss caused by experimental periodontitis in monkeys. J Periodont Res 1994; 29: 35–40.

118. Yaffe A., Fine N., Alt I. & Binderman I. The effect of bisphosphonate on alveolar bone resorption following mucoperiosteal flap surgery in the mandible of rats. J Periodontol 1995; 66: 999–1003.

119. Shoji K., Horiuchi H. & ShinodaH. Inhibitory effects of a bisphosphonate (risedronate) on experimental periodontitis in rats. J Periodont Res 1995; 30: 277–284.

120. Yaffe A., Iztkovich Y., Earon I., Lilov R. & Binderman I. Local delivery of an amino bisphosphonate prevents the resorptive phase of alveolar bone following mucoperiosteal flap surgery in rats. J Periodontol 1997; 68: 884–889.

121. Ouchi N., Nishikawa H., Yoshino T., Kanoh H., Motoie H., Nishimori E., Shimaoka T., Abe T., Shikama H., Fujikura T., Matsue M. & Matsue I. Inhibitory effects of YM175, a bisphosphonate, on the progression of experimental periodontitis in beagle dogs. J Periodont Res 1998; 33:196–204.

122. Binderman I., Adut M. & Yaffe A. Effectiveness of local delivery of alendronate in reducing alveolar bone loss following periodontal surgery in rats. J Periodontol 2000; 71: 1236–1240.

123. Alencar V. B. M., Bezzerra M. M., Lima V. Abreu A. L. C., Brito G. A. C., Rocha F. A. C. & Ribeiro R. A. Disodium chlodronate prevents bone resorption in experimental periodontitis in rats. J Periodontol 2002; 73: 251–256.

124. Kaynak D., Meffert R., Bostanci H. A histopathological investigation on the effect of systemic administration of the bisphosphonate alendronate on resorptive phase following mucoperiosteal flap surgery in the rat mandible. J Periodontol 2003; 74:1348–1354.

125. Takaishi Y., Ikeo T., Miki T., Nishizawa Y. & Morii H. Suppression of alveolar bone resorption by etidronate treatment for periodontal disease: 4-to 5-year follow-up of four patients. Cited by Salvi GE, Lang NP. Host response modulation in the management of periodontal diseases in J Clin Peridontol 2005; 32 (Suppl. 6): 108–129.

126. Rocha ML, Malcara JM, Sanchez-Martin FJ, Vazquez de la Torre CJ, Fajardo ME. Effects of alendronate on periodontal disease in postmenopausal women: a randomized placebo-controlled trial. J Periodontol 2004; 75:1579-1585.

127. MH.Parker, Maurizio T.Gene expression profile of periodontal ligament cells treated with enamel matrix proteins in vitro:analysis with cDNA arrays.J.Periodontol,2004:75;1539-1546.

128. Lane N, Gary C. Armitage, Peter Loomer, Susan Hsieh, Sharmila Majumdar, H.-Y. Wang, Marjorie, and Thelma Munoz. Bisphosphonate Therapy Improves the Outcome of Conventional Periondontal Treatment: Results of a 12-Month, Randomized, Placebo-Controlled Study. J Periodontol 2005; 76:1113-1122.

129. J.Goya, H.Paez. Effect of topical application of monosodium olpadronate on experimental periodontitis in rats.J.Periodontol,2006;77:1-6.

130. Gabriela Geiro, CE.Sakakura.Efffect of 17βesteradiol & alendronate on temoval torque of osseointegrated titanium implants in ovariectomized rats.J.Periodontol,2007;78:1316-1321.

131. Palmo.L, Bissada NF. Skeletal bone diseases impact the periodontium: a review of bisphosphonate therapy. Expert Opin pharmacotherapy; 2007Feb 8(3):309-15.

132. Qiming Jin,J. Cerilli. RANKL inhibition through osteoprotegrin blocks bone loss in experimental periodontitis. J. Periodontol,2007;78:1300-1308.

133. Sunao Sato, M.Kitagawa. Enamel Matrix Derivative Exhibits Anti-Inflammatory Properties in Monocytes. J. Periodontol,2008;79:535-540.

134. Noguchi, K., Shitashige, M., Endo, H., Kondo, H., Yotsumoto, Y., Izumi, Y., Nitta, H. & Ishikawa, I. Involvement of cyclooxygenase- 2 in serum-induced prostaglandin production by human oral gingival epithelial cells. J Periodont Res 2001; 36: 124–130.

135. Noguchi, K., Shitashige, M., Endo, H., Kondo, H., Yotsumoto, Y., Izumi, Y., Nitta, H. & Ishikawa, I. Involvement of cyclooxygenase- 2 in serum- induced prostaglandin production by human oral gingival epithelial cells. J Periodont Res 2001; 36: 124–130.

136. Buduneli, N., Vardar, S., Atilla, G., Sorsa, T.,Luoto, H. & Baylas, H. Gingival crevicular fluid matrix metalloproteinase-8 levels following adjunctive use of meloxicam and initial phase of periodontal therapy. J Periodontol 2002; 73:103–109.

137. Hawkey C. J. Gastroduodenal problems associated with non- steroidal anti-inflammatory drugs (NSAIDs). Cited by Salvi GE, Lang NP. Host response modulation in the management of periodontal diseases in J Clin Peridontol 2005; 32 (Suppl. 6): 108–129.

138. Lindsley C. & Warady, B. Non-steroidal anti-inflammatory drugs. Renal toxicity. Review of perdiatric issues. Cited by Salvi GE, Lang NP. Host response modulation in the management of periodontal diseases in J Clin Peridontol 2005; 32 (Suppl. 6): 108–129.

139. Wardle E. N. COX-2 inhibitors and risk of heart failure. Cited by Salvi GE, Lang NP. Host response modulation in the management of periodontal diseases in J Clin Peridontol 2005; 32 (Suppl. 6): 108–129.

140. Van Dyke TE. & Serhan, C. N. Resolution of inflammation: a new paradigm for the pathogenesis of periodontal diseases. J Dent Res 2003; 82. 82–90.

141. Claria J, Serhan CN. Aspirin triggers previously undescribed bioactive eicosanoids by human endothelial cell-leukocyte interactions. Cited by Alpdogan Kantarci, Thomas E. Van Dyke. Lipoxins in Chronic Inflammation in Crit Rev Oral Biol Med 2003; 14(1):4-12.

142. Pouliot M, Clish CB, Petasis NA, Van Dyke TE, Serhan CN. Lipoxin A4 analogues inhibit leukocyte recruitment to *Porphyromonas gingivalis*: a role for cyclooxygenase-2 and lipoxins in periodontal disease. Cited by Alpdogan Kantarci, Thomas E. Van Dyke. Lipoxins in Chronic Inflammation in Crit Rev Oral Biol Med 2003; 14(1):4-12.

143. Ryan ME, Ramamurthy S, Golub LM. Matrix metalloproteinases and their inhibition in periodontal treatment. Cited by Preshaw PM, Hefti AF, Jepsen S, Etienne D, Walker C, Bradshaw MH Subantimicrobial dose doxycycline as adjunctive treatment for periodontitis in J Clin Periodontol 2004; 31: 697–707.

144. Gordon J, Walker C, Murphy J, Goodson J, Socransky S. Tetracycline: Levels achievable in gingival crevice fluid and *in vitro* effect on subgingival microorganisms. I. Concentrations in crevicular fluid after repeated doses. J Periodontol 1981: **52**: 609–612.

145. Pascale D, Gordon J, Lamster I, Mann P, Seiger M, Arndt W. Concentration of doxycycline in human gingival fluid. J Clin Periodontol 1986: 13: 841–844.

146. Golub LM., Lee, H. M., Ryan, M. E., Giannobile, W. V., Payne, J. & Sorsa, T. Tetracyclines inhibit connective tissue breakdown by multiple non-antimicrobial actions. Cited by Preshaw PM, Hefti AF, Jepsen S,

Etienne D, Walker C, Bradshaw MH Subantimicrobial dose doxycycline as adjunctive treatment for periodontitis in J Clin Periodontol 2004; 31: 697–707.

147. Burns FR., Stack, M. S., Gray, R. D. & Paterson, C. A. Inhibition of purified collagenase from alkali-burned rabbit corneas. Cited by Preshaw PM, Hefti AF, Jepsen S, Etienne D, Walker C, Bradshaw MH Subantimicrobial dose doxycycline as adjunctive treatment for periodontitis in J Clin Periodontol 2004; 31: 697–707.

148. Smith GN. Jr., Mickler, E. A., Hasty, K. A. & Brandt, K. D. Specificity of inhibition of matrix metalloproteinase activity by doxycycline: relationship to structure of the enzyme. Cited by Preshaw PM, Hefti AF, Jepsen S, Etienne D, Walker C, Bradshaw MH Subantimicrobial dose doxycycline as adjunctive treatment for periodontitis in J Clin Periodontol 2004; 31: 697–707.

149. Preshaw PM, Hefti AF, Jepsen S, Etienne D, Walker C, Bradshaw MH Subantimicrobial dose doxycycline as adjunctive treatment for periodontitis A review: J Clin Periodontol 2004; 31: 697–707.

150. Ryan ME. & Ashley, R. A. How do tetracyclines work? Cited by Preshaw PM, Hefti AF, Jepsen S, Etienne D, Walker C, Bradshaw MH Subantimicrobial dose doxycycline as adjunctive treatment for periodontitis in J Clin Periodontol 2004; 31: 697–707.

151. Nagase H, Itoh, Y. & Binner, S. (1994) Interaction of alpha 2-macroglobulin with matrix metalloproteinases and its use for identification of their active forms. Cited by Salvi GE, Lang NP. Host

response modulation in the management of periodontal diseases in J Clin Peridontol 2005; 32 (Suppl. 6): 108–129.

152. Rifkin BR, Vernillo, A. T., Golub, L. M. & Ramamurthy, N. S. Modulation of bone resorption by tetracyclines. Cited by Salvi GE, Lang NP. Host response modulation in the management of periodontal diseases in J Clin Peridontol 2005; 32 (Suppl. 6): 108–129.

153. Uitto VJ., Firth, J. D., Nip, L. & Golub, L. M(1994). Doxycycline and chemically modified tetracyclines inhibit gelatinase A (MMP-2) gene expression in human skin keratinocytes. Cited by Preshaw PM, Hefti AF, Jepsen S, Etienne D, Walker C, Bradshaw MH Subantimicrobial dose doxycycline as adjunctive treatment for periodontitis in J Clin Periodontol 2004; 31: 697–707.

154. Milano S, Arcoleo, F., D'Agostino, P. & Cillari, E. Intraperitoneal injection of tetracyclines protects mice from lethal endotoxemia downregulating inducible nitric oxide synthase in various organs and cytokine and nitrate secretion in blood. Cited by Salvi GE, Lang NP. Host response modulation in the management of periodontal diseases in J Clin Peridontol 2005; 32 (Suppl. 6): 108–129.

155. Preshaw PM., Hefti, A. F., Novak, M. J.,Michalowicz, B. S., Pihlstrom, B. L., Schoor, R., Trummel, C. L., Dean, J., Van Dyke, T. E., Walker, C. B. & Bradshaw, M. H. Subantimicrobial dose doxycycline enhances the efficacy of scaling and root planing in chronic periodontitis: a multicenter trial. J Periodontol 2004; 75:1068–1076.

156. Teronen O., Heikkila P., Konttinen Y. T., Laitinen M., Salo T., Hanemaaijer R., Teronen A., Maisi P. & Sorsa T. MMP inhibition and downregulation by bisphosphonates. Cited by Salvi GE, Lang NP. Host response modulation in the management of periodontal diseases in J Clin Peridontol 2005; 32 (Suppl. 6): 108–129.

157. Galardy R, Grobelny D, Kortylewicz Z, Poncz L. Inhibition of human skin fibroblast collagenase by phosphorus-containing peptides. Cited by Maria Emanuel Ryan & Lorne M. Golub Modulation of matrix metalloproteinase activities in periodontitis as a treatment strategy in Periodontol 2000, Vol. 24, 2000, 226–238.

158. Schwartz M, Venkataraman S, Libby A, Mookhtiar K, Mallya S, Van Wart H, Birkedal-Hansen H. Sulfur-based inihibitors for matrix metalloproteinases. Cited by Maria Emanuel Ryan & Lorne M. Golub Modulation of matrix metalloproteinase activities in periodontitis as a treatment strategy in Periodontol 2000, Vol. 24, 2000, 226–238.

159. Nagai Y, Hattori S, Odake S, Okayama T, Obata M, Morikawa T. Preparation of peptidyl hydroxamic acid derivatives which inhibit interstitial collagenases. Cited by Maria Emanuel Ryan & Lorne M. Golub Modulation of matrix metalloproteinase activities in periodontitis as a treatment strategy in Periodontol 2000, Vol. 24, 2000, 226–238.

160. Hudson BI. & Schmidt, A. M. RAGE: a novel target for drug intervention in diabetic vascular disease. Cited by Salvi GE, Lang NP. Host response modulation in the management of periodontal diseases in J Clin Peridontol 2005; 32 (Suppl. 6): 108–129.

161. Hudson BI., Bucciarelli, L. G., Wendt, T., Sakaguchi, T., Lalla, E., Qu, W., Lu, Y., Lee, L., Stern, D. M., Naka, Y., Ramasamy, R., Yan, S. D., Yan, S. F., D&aposAgati, V. & Schmidt, A. M. Blockade of receptor for advanced glycation endproducts: a new target for therapeutic intervention in diabetic complications and inflammatory disorders. Cited by Salvi GE, Lang NP. Host response modulation in the management of periodontal diseases in J Clin Peridontol 2005; 32 (Suppl. 6): 108–129.

162. Vlassara H, Brownlee, M., Manogue, K. R., Dinarello, C. A. & Pasagian, A. Cachectin/TNF and IL-1 induced by glucose- modified proteins: role in normal tissue remodeling. Cited by Salvi GE, Lang NP. Host response modulation in the management of periodontal diseases in J Clin Peridontol 2005; 32 (Suppl. 6): 108–129.

163. Lalla E, Lamster IB., Feit M, Huang L., Spessot A., Qu W, Kislinger, TY, Stern D. M. & Schmidt A. M. Blockade of RAGE suppresses periodontitis-associated bone loss in diabetic mice. Cited by Salvi GE, Lang NP. Host response modulation in the management of periodontal diseases in J Clin Peridontol 2005; 32 (Suppl. 6): 108–129.

164. Killborn RG, Belloni P. endothelial cell proliferation of nitrogen oxides in response to interferon gamma in combination with tumor necrosis factor, interleukin-1, or endotoxin. Cited by Daghigh, F., Borghaei, R. C., Thornton, R. D. & Bee, J. H. Human gingival fibroblasts produce nitric oxide in response to proinflammatory cytokines in J Periodontol 2002; 73, 392–400.

165. al-Ramadi BK, Meissler JJ Jr, Huang D, Eisenstein TK. Immunosuppression induced by nitric oxide and its inhibition by

interleukin-4. Cited by Daghigh, F., Borghaei, R. C., Thornton, R. D. & Bee, J. H. Human gingival fibroblasts produce nitric oxide in response to proinflammatory cytokines in J Periodontol 2002; 73, 392–400.

166. Zingarelli B., Southan, G. J., Gilad, E., O'Connor, M., Salzman, A. L. & Szabo, C. The inhibitory effects of mercaptoalkylguanidines on cyclo-oxygenase activity. Cited by Salvi GE, Lang NP. Host response modulation in the management of periodontal diseases in J Clin Peridontol 2005; 32 (Suppl. 6): 108–129.

167. Szabo C., Ferrer-Sueta, G., Zingarelli, B., Southan, G. J., Salzman, A. L. & Radi, R. Mercaptoethylguanidine and guanidine inhibitors of nitric oxide synthase react with peroxynitrite and protect against peroxynitrite-induced oxidative damage. Cited by Salvi GE, Lang NP. Host response modulation in the management of periodontal diseases in J Clin Peridontol 2005; 32 (Suppl. 6): 108–129.

168. Esposito M, Grusovin MG. Enamel matrix derivative (Emdogain) for periodontal tissue regeneration in intrabony defects.Cochrane database Syst Rev 2005 ;(4):CD003875.

169. Simonet WS., Lacey, D. L., Dunstan, C. R., Kelley, M., Chang, M. S., Luthy, R., Nguyen, H. Q., Wooden, S., Bennett, L., Boone, T., Shimamoto, G., DeRose, M., Elliott, R., Colombero, A., Tan, H. L., Train, G., Sullivan, J., Davy, E., Bucay, N., Renshaw-Gegg, L., Hughes, T. M., Hill, D., Pattison, W., Campell, P. & Boyle W, . J. Osteoprotegerin: a novel secreted protein involved in the regulation of bone density. Cited by Keith L. Kirkwood, Joni A. Cirelli, Jill E. Rogers and Williams V.

Giannobile. Novel Host Response Therapeutic Approaches to treat periodontal diseases in Periodontol 2000. Vol 43; 2007; 294-315.

170. Mahamed DA, Marleau A, Alnaeeli M, Singh B, Zhang X, Penninger JM, Teng YT. G(-) anaerobes-reactive CD4+ T-cells trigger RANKL-mediated enhanced alveolar bone loss in diabetic NOD mice. Cited by Keith L. Kirkwood, Joni A. Cirelli, Jill E. Rogers and Williams V. Giannobile. Novel Host Response Therapeutic Approaches to treat periodontal diseases in Periodontol 2000. Vol 43; 2007; 294-315.

171. Rogers MJ., Gordon S., Benford H. L., Coxon F. P., Luckman S. P., Monkkonen J. & Frith J. C. Cellular and molecular mechanisms of action of bisphosphonates. Cited by Keith L. Kirkwood, Joni A. Cirelli, Jill E. Rogers and Williams V. Giannobile. Novel Host Response Therapeutic Approaches to treat periodontal diseases in Periodontol 2000. Vol 43; 2007; 294-315.

172. Fleisch H. Bisphosphonates: mechanisms of action and clinical use in osteoporosis- an update. Cited by Salvi GE, Lang NP. Host response modulation in the management of periodontal diseases in J Clin Peridontol 2005; 32 (Suppl. 6): 108–129.

173. Reddy MS., Weatherford TW. III, Smith C. A., West B. D., Jeffcoat M K. & Jacks T. M. Alendronate treatment of naturally-occurring periodontitis in beagle dogs. J Periodontol 1995; 66:211–217.

174. Robert J Genco. Clinical innovations in managing inflammation & periodontal diseases: The workshop on inflammation & periodontal diseases. J.Periodontol, 2008, Vol. 79, No. 8s, Pages 1609-1611.